THE ULTIMATE EXERCISE GUIDE: ABDOMINALS EDITION

152 HOW-TO INSTRUCTIONS FOR HOME AND GYM
1ST EDITION

PUBLISHER: N.C.A. HEALTH & WELLNESS
AUTHOR: NICOLAS ANDREOU

Disclaimer

The information in this book is provided for educational and informational purposes only and is not intended as medical advice. The fitness exercises described are intended for healthy individuals without any medical conditions or injuries that could be aggravated by physical activity.

While every effort has been made to ensure the accuracy and clarity of the exercise descriptions and illustrations, the nature of 3D designs and illustrations may introduce variations or inaccuracies. These visuals are only meant to guide proper form and technique but may not fully represent every individual's unique anatomy or movement pattern. Users are encouraged to prioritize safety, use proper judgment, and seek professional guidance when necessary.

The author and publisher are not responsible for any injury, accident, or health complication that may arise from applying the exercises and information in this book. Use of the information is at your own risk.

Before beginning any exercise program, you should consult with your physician or other health care professional to ensure that the exercises are appropriate for your specific health condition, especially if you have a history of injury, surgery, or any medical condition. Participation in any exercise program may result in injury. By voluntarily engaging in these exercises, you assume the risk of any resulting injury and accept full responsibility for your health and safety.

Neither the author, **Nicolas Andreou**, nor **N.C.A. HEALTH & WELLNESS LTD** shall be held liable or responsible for any injury, loss, or damage arising from this book or the reliance on any information contained within it. Use of the exercises and advice in this book is at your own risk.

The mention and depiction of gym and fitness equipment within this book, including but not limited to barbells, dumbbells, resistance bands, machines, and other equipment, are intended solely for descriptive and instructional purposes. Any similarities to specific brands, models, or proprietary designs are purely coincidental and are used under the principles of **fair use**. The equipment depicted is intended to represent general types of fitness tools commonly available, and no endorsement or affiliation with any specific manufacturer is implied.

CONTENTS

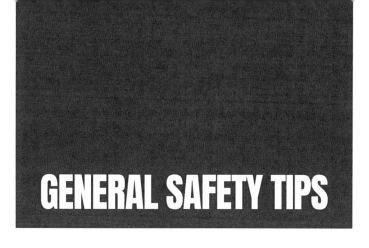

GENERAL SAFETY TIPS

Always prioritize safety when exercising, mainly when using weights or resistance equipment. Following proper safety guidelines will help you maximize your workout results and minimize the risk of injury.

1. **Warm Up Properly:** Always start your workout with a proper warm-up to prepare your muscles, joints, and cardiovascular system for exercise. Spend 5-10 minutes doing light aerobic exercises (like jogging or cycling) and dynamic stretches to increase blood flow and loosen tight muscles.

2. **Focus on Proper Form:** Performing exercises with the correct form is crucial for effectiveness and safety. Pay close attention to your body alignment and movement. If unsure about your form, consider using mirrors or asking a fitness professional to review your technique. Don't sacrifice form for heavier weights.

3. **Start with Lighter Weights:** If you're new to strength training or a specific exercise, start with lighter weights to master the movement before progressing to heavier loads. Gradual progression helps build strength safely, preventing strain or injury to muscles, joints, and ligaments.

4. **Use Controlled Movements:** Avoid fast, jerky movements that can increase the risk of injury. Instead, focus on slow, controlled motions, particularly during the eccentric phase (lowering the weight). Control ensures that the muscles are

doing the work, not momentum, and reduces strain on your joints.

5. **Breathe Properly:** Breathing is an often-overlooked aspect of training. Exhale during the exertion phase (the most challenging part of the exercise) and inhale during the relaxation phase. Proper breathing supports your muscles and helps maintain stable blood pressure.

6. **Don't Overtrain:** Your muscles need time to recover and grow. Overtraining without adequate rest increases the risk of fatigue-related injuries and hinders progress. Allow at least 48 hours of rest before working the same muscle group again.

7. **Listen to Your Body:** If you experience any sharp pain, dizziness, or discomfort, stop immediately. Pain is your body's way of telling you something isn't right. Rest, assess the situation, and, if needed, consult a healthcare professional before resuming.

8. **Cool Down and Stretch:** Finish your workout with a proper cool-down. Gentle stretching and light activity help reduce muscle stiffness, prevent injury, and promote flexibility. This ensures a gradual return to your normal heart rate and prevents post-exercise soreness.

SUPPORTING OUR WORK AND GROWTH

At **ExerciseAnimatic.com**, we're committed to continuously expanding our exercise library, producing new videos, and offering high-quality resources to help you reach your fitness goals. We're passionate about providing tools that support your progress and make your fitness journey more engaging and effective.

If you'd like to support our ongoing efforts, you can scan the following QR code to explore the **Ultimate Bundle** on our website. This lifetime-access bundle includes 1650+ exercise videos, perfectly complementing the exercises in this book, offering visual demonstrations that guide your technique and form.

Additionally, using the code **'IBOUGHTYOURBOOK'**, you can receive a **20% discount** on your first order, whether it's the Ultimate Bundle or individual exercise videos that complement your workout routine. Every purchase helps us produce new content, expand our library, and provide valuable resources to the fitness community.

Thank you for being part of our journey and supporting us as we strive to bring more innovative fitness content to individuals like you. Your support allows us to keep growing and creating resources that empower people to live healthier, stronger lives.

CHAPTER 1

INTRODUCTION

Building a strong and well-defined core isn't just about aesthetics—it's about enhancing your body's stability, strength, and overall functional fitness. Whether you're an experienced athlete fine-tuning your ab routine or a beginner aiming to develop core strength, *The Ultimate Exercise Guide: Abdominals Edition* is your go-to resource for achieving your goals.

With 152 carefully selected exercises, this book is more than just a guide—it's a complete resource designed to help you master abdominal development for both functional strength and definition. I wrote this book to provide a detailed, step-by-step approach to working out your abdominals, whether at home, in the gym, or on the move.

Why Focus on Abdominals?

The abdominals, often referred to as the core, are a crucial muscle group responsible for stability, posture, and overall body strength. They are engaged every time you twist, bend, or stabilize your torso. Strong abdominals are essential for building a balanced and powerful physique, as they support everyday functional movements and enhance your performance in exercises like squats, deadlifts, and any activity requiring balance. Dedicating time to abdominal training improves your appearance and strengthens your core, making everyday movements and gym exercises more efficient and effective.

Why This Book is Different

The Ultimate Exercise Guide: Abdominals Edition stands out from other fitness guides for its focus on versatility and accessibility. Whether you are just starting your fitness journey or an experienced athlete, this book offers a wide range of exercises tailored to your needs. It covers everything from beginner-friendly core exercises to advanced variations designed to push even the most seasoned athletes. With options for bodyweight and equipment-based workouts, this guide ensures you can strengthen and sculpt your abdominals regardless of your environment or fitness level.

With this edition, you'll have access to:

✦ **152 Abdominal Exercises**: Covering bodyweight movements, dumbbells, cables, resistance bands, machines, and more, we ensure there's something for everyone.

✦ **Clear, Detailed Instructions**: Each exercise is broken down step by step so you can focus on proper form and execution.

✦ **High-Quality Illustrations**: Visuals accompany every exercise to ensure you perform movements safely and effectively.

✦ **Home and Gym Adaptations**: Whether working out in a fully equipped gym or your living room, you'll find exercises that fit your space and tools.

✦ **Tips**: Important tips to help you perform the exercises safely and effectively for a complete workout experience.

How to Use This Book

The guide is structured in a simple and effective way to help you quickly find exercises based on your available equipment. The exercises are grouped by equipment type - bodyweight, dumbbells, resistance bands, and more - so you can quickly navigate to the section that fits your current workout environment.

For each exercise, you'll find:

✦ **A detailed description** of how to perform the movement safely and correctly.

✦ **Active muscle engagement**, so you know exactly what you're working on.

✦ **Important tips** to help you avoid injury and make the most out of every rep.

✦ **QR codes link to videos** that offer visual demonstrations of every exercise. Scan the codes with your phone camera, and the demonstration of each exercise will automatically pop up on your screen.

Your Abdominals Transformation Starts Here

Strong, well-defined abdominal muscles are not just about aesthetics but also about enhancing your overall core strength, stability, and athletic performance. By dedicating time to training your abdominals, you are laying the foundation for better posture, improved balance, and more efficient movements in everyday activities and workouts.

This book is designed to be your go-to reference—a guide you can revisit as you progress in your fitness journey. It's a tool to help you unlock your potential, challenge your limits, and achieve solid results.

Whether you're just beginning or looking to elevate your ab workout routine, *The Ultimate Exercise Guide: Abdominals Edition* will equip you with the exercises, knowledge, and confidence to succeed. Let's dive in and start building a stronger core, one rep at a time.

CHAPTER 2

BODYWEIGHT EXERCISES

What Are Bodyweight Exercises?

Bodyweight exercises are physical movements that rely solely on your own body weight to provide resistance, rather than using external equipment like dumbbells or machines. These exercises typically involve pushing, pulling, or lifting your body against gravity and simultaneously engaging multiple muscle groups. Common bodyweight exercises include push-ups, squats, lunges, and planks. Because they don't require equipment, bodyweight exercises can be performed anywhere, making them accessible for all fitness levels and adaptable to various workout routines.

Why Use Bodyweight Exercises?

Bodyweight exercises offer several benefits, making them an excellent addition to any fitness program. They improve strength, flexibility, and endurance while promoting functional movement, which helps improve everyday activities. Since these exercises engage stabilizing muscles, they also help to improve balance and coordination. Additionally, bodyweight exercises are ideal for beginners and advanced athletes, as they can be easily modified to increase or decrease intensity. Whether at home, traveling, or in a gym, bodyweight exercises provide a convenient, effective, and versatile way to stay fit.

1. 3-4 Sit-Up

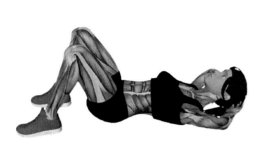

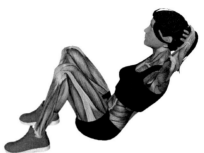

Instructions:

1. Lie on your back with your knees bent and your feet flat on the floor, hip-width apart.

2. Place your hands behind your head, keeping your elbows wide.

3. Engage your core and lift your upper body towards your knees, coming up about three-quarters of the way.

4. Slowly lower your upper body back to the starting position and repeat.

Tips:

1. Keep your core engaged throughout the exercise to avoid straining your lower back.

2. Avoid pulling on your neck with your hands; use your abdominal muscles to lift your upper body.

3. Breathe steadily, exhaling as you lift and inhaling as you lower.

Active Muscles:
Primary: Abdominals (Rectus Abdominis)
Secondary: Hip Flexors (Iliopsoas)

Equipment:
None

2. 45 Degree Bicycle Twisting

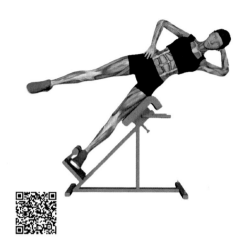

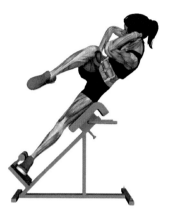

Instructions:

1. Align yourself to 45 degrees to the floor by fixing your left foot into the footrest and supporting your thigh against the Hyperextension bench.

2. Place your left hand behind your head and your right hand on your waist.

3. Open your upper leg slightly and bend your knee while bringing your opposite elbow towards it.

4. Return to the initial position and repeat.

Tips:

1. Keep your hips pressed on the hyperextension bench to engage your core muscles more effectively and protect your spine.

2. Avoid pulling on your neck with your hand; use your core to lift and twist, keeping your neck in a neutral position.

3. Perform the exercise slowly and deliberately to maximize muscle engagement and reduce the risk of strain.

Active Muscles:
Primary: Obliques (external and internal obliques)
Secondary: Abdominals (rectus abdominis)

Equipment:
Hyperextension Bench

3. 45 Degree Side Bend

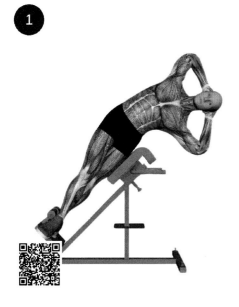

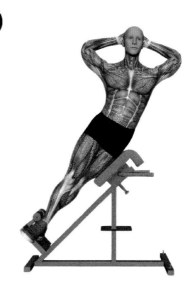

Instructions:
1. Place your feet one after the other onto the footrests and support your thigh against the Hyperextension Platform.
2. Place your hands behind your head and assume a position with a straight back.
3. Crunch your torso toward the floor and then upwards.
4. Repeat while keeping yourself stable on the bench.

Tips:
1. Maintain a steady and controlled pace to ensure proper form and prevent strain.
2. Focus on using your oblique muscles to lift your upper body, avoiding any jerking or sudden movements.
3. Keep your neck in a neutral position to avoid straining it during the exercise.

Active Muscles:
Primary: Obliques (external and internal obliques)
Secondary: Abdominals (rectus abdominis), Lower Back (erector spinae)

Equipment:
Hyperextension Bench

4. 45 Degree Twisting Hyperextension

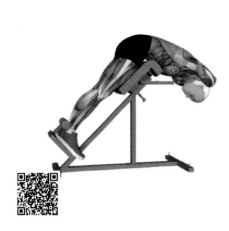

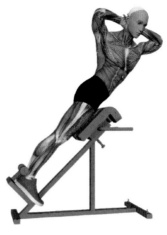

Instructions:
1. Fix your feet to the footrests and press your thighs against the padded platform of a Hyperextension Bench.
2. Place your hands behind your head and lean down to the floor, keeping your back straight.
3. Raise yourself by extending backward and twisting your torso to the side.
4. Hold for a second, return to the initial position, and repeat.

Tips:
1. Perform the twisting motion smoothly and avoid jerking to prevent strain on your back.
2. Engage your core muscles throughout the exercise to maintain stability and support your spine.
3. Breathe steadily, exhaling as you lift and twist, and inhaling as you lower back down.

Active Muscles:
Primary: Lower Back (erector spinae), Obliques (external and internal obliques)
Secondary: Abdominals (rectus abdominis), Glutes (gluteus maximus)

Equipment:
Hyperextension Bench

5. 90 Degree Heel Touch

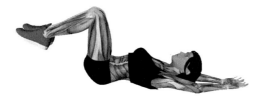

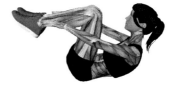

Instructions:

1. Lie down on your back with your hips and knees bent to 90 degrees and your arms extended overhead.

2. Raise your upper back and bring your arms forward to touch your heels.

3. Hold for a second, return to the initial position, and repeat.

Tips:

1. Keep your neck relaxed and avoid straining it by using your core muscles to lift your shoulders.

2. Ensure your lower back stays pressed into the floor or mat to engage your core effectively and protect your spine.

3. Perform the exercise with controlled movements to maximize muscle engagement and reduce the risk of injury.

Active Muscles:
Primary: Abdominals (rectus abdominis)
Secondary: Hip Flexors (iliopsoas)

Equipment:
None

6. Ab Mat Sit-Up

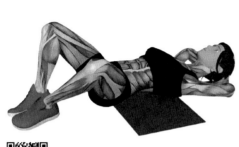 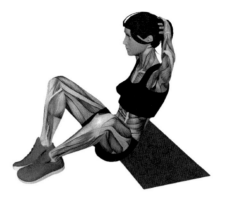

Instructions:

1. Sit on the floor with a yoga mat placed under your lower back, knees bent facing outwards, and feet on the floor touching together. Place your hands behind your head.

2. Lean back to lie down, keeping your arms behind your head.

3. Use your core muscles to sit your torso up, return to the starting position and repeat.

Tips:

1. Focus on your core muscles throughout the movement to maximize effectiveness and protect your lower back.

2. Avoid using momentum by performing the movement slowly and with control.

3. Keep your feet together and your knees stable to maintain proper form.

Active Muscles:
Primary: Abdominals (rectus abdominis)
Secondary: Hip Flexors (iliopsoas), Adductors

Equipment:
Yoga/Exercise Mat

7. Ab Tuck

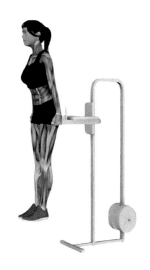

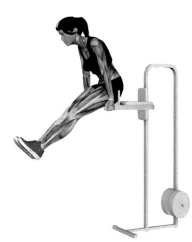

Instructions:

1. Start by hanging on a dip station, holding the parallel bars with your arms extended and your body straight.
2. Lift your knees towards your chest while lightly extending your hips backward, engaging your core muscles.
3. Extend your legs back downwards to the starting position.
4. Repeat the movement.

Tips:

1. Engage your core muscles throughout the exercise to maintain control and stability.
2. Perform the movement slowly and deliberately to avoid using momentum and maximize muscle engagement.
3. Keep your upper body stable and avoid swinging to ensure proper form.

Active Muscles:
Primary: Abdominals (rectus abdominis)
Secondary: Hip Flexors (iliopsoas), Quadriceps (Quadriceps Femoris)

Equipment:
Dip Station

8. Abdominal Crunches

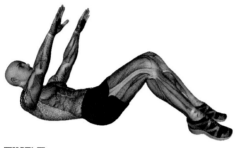

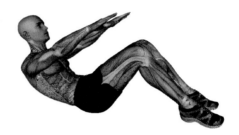

Instructions:

1. Lie on your back with knees bent, feet placed flat on the floor, and arms raised straight to shoulder height upwards.

2. Squeeze your abdominals to lift your upper back off the floor, reaching forward with your arms.

3. Hold for a second, slowly return to the starting position and repeat.

Tips:

1. Keep your neck relaxed and avoid stressing it during exercise to prevent strain.

2. Focus on engaging your core muscles throughout the movement to maximize effectiveness.

3. Breathe steadily, exhaling as you lift into the crunch and inhaling as you lower back down.

Active Muscles:
Primary: Abdominals (rectus abdominis)
Secondary: Obliques (external and internal obliques)

Equipment:
None

9. Air Bike (VERSION 2)

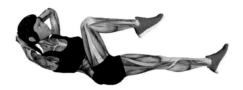

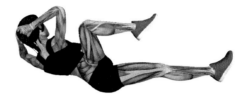

Instructions:
1. Lie on your back with your hands behind your head and your knees bent at a 90-degree angle.
2. Lift your shoulders off the floor, engaging your core.
3. Bring your right elbow towards your left knee while extending your right leg straight.
4. Switch sides, bringing your left elbow towards your right knee while extending your left leg straight. Continue alternating sides in a pedaling motion.

Tips:
5. Keep your core engaged throughout the exercise to maximize muscle activation and protect your lower back.
6. Perform the movement slowly and with control, avoiding the use of momentum to maximize effectiveness.
7. Breathe steadily, exhaling as you twist and bring your elbow to your knee, and inhaling as you switch sides.

Active Muscles:
Primary: Abdominals (rectus abdominis), Obliques (external and internal obliques)

Secondary: Hip Flexors (iliopsoas), Quadriceps (quadriceps femoris)
Equipment:
None

10. Air Bike

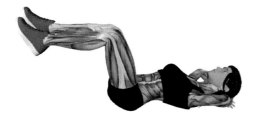

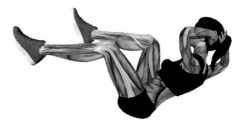

Instructions:

1. Lie on your back with your hands behind your head and your knees bent at a 90-degree angle.

2. Lift your back off the floor, engaging your core.

3. Bring your right elbow towards your left knee while extending your right leg slightly.

4. Lower your back to the floor and repeat, bringing your left elbow towards your right knee while extending your left leg lightly.

Tips:

1. Keep your core engaged throughout the exercise to maximize muscle activation and protect your lower back.

2. Perform the movement slowly and with control, avoiding the use of momentum to maximize effectiveness.

3. Breathe steadily, exhaling as you twist and bring your elbow to your knee, and inhaling as you switch sides.

Active Muscles:
Primary: Abdominals (rectus abdominis), Obliques (external and internal obliques)

Secondary: Hip Flexors (iliopsoas), Quadriceps (quadriceps femoris)
Equipment:
None

11. Air Twisting Crunch

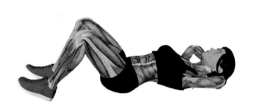

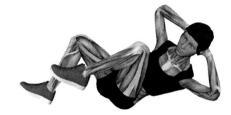

Instructions:

1. Lie down on your back with your knees bent and heels on the floor.

2. Place your hands behind your head.

3. Raise your chest and twist your torso to one side while bringing the opposite knee close.

4. Return to the initial position and repeat by twisting towards the other side.

Tips:

1. Keep your core engaged throughout the exercise to maximize muscle activation and protect your lower back.

2. Perform the movement slowly and with control, avoiding the use of momentum to maximize effectiveness.

3. Breathe steadily, exhaling as you twist and bring your elbow to your knee, and inhaling as you switch sides.

Active Muscles:

Primary: Abdominals (rectus abdominis), Obliques (external and internal obliques)

Secondary: Hip Flexors (iliopsoas), Quadriceps (quadriceps femoris)

Equipment:

None

12. Alternate Arm Leg Plank Hold

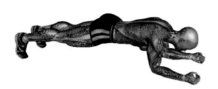
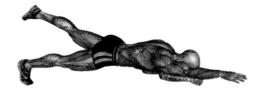

Instructions:

1. Start in a plank position with your elbows directly under your shoulders and your body forming a straight line from head to heels.

2. Lift your right arm and left leg simultaneously, extending them straight out while maintaining balance. Hold this position for a brief period of 5 seconds.

3. Lower your right arm and left leg back to the plank position.

4. Lift your left arm and right leg simultaneously, extending them straight out and holding for a brief period of 5 seconds before returning to the plank position.

Tips:

1. Keep your core engaged throughout the exercise to maintain stability and prevent your hips from sagging.

2. Perform the movement slowly and with control to maximize muscle engagement and maintain balance.

3. Breathe steadily, exhaling as you lift your arm and leg and inhaling as you hold the position.

Active Muscles:
Primary: Core Muscles (rectus abdominis, obliques)

Secondary: Glutes (gluteus maximus)

Equipment:
None

13. Alternate Arm Leg Plank

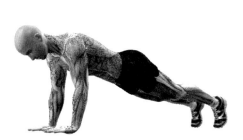
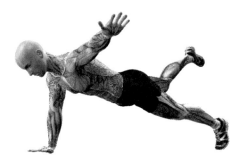

Instructions:
1. Start in a plank position with your hands directly under your shoulders and your body forming a straight line from head to heels.
2. Lift your right arm and left leg simultaneously, extending them straight out while maintaining balance. Hold for a second, then lower back to the plank position.
3. Lift your left arm and right leg simultaneously, extending them straight out and holding for a second before returning to the plank position.
4. Continue alternating sides, lifting opposite arms and legs.

Tips:
1. Keep your core engaged throughout the exercise to maintain stability and prevent your hips from sagging.
2. Perform the movement slowly and with control to maximize muscle engagement and maintain balance.
3. Breathe steadily, exhaling as you lift your arm and leg and inhaling as you lower them back to the plank position.

Active Muscles:
Primary: Core Muscles (rectus abdominis, obliques), Shoulders (deltoids)

Secondary: Glutes (gluteus maximus)

Equipment:
None

14. Alternate Heel Touches

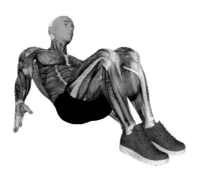
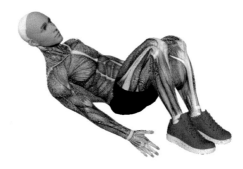

Instructions:

1. Lie on your back with your knees bent and feet flat on the floor, hip-width apart. Lift your shoulders slightly off the floor, engaging your core.

2. Reach your right hand towards your right heel, then return to the center position.

3. Reach your left hand towards your left heel.

4. Continue alternating sides for the required repetitions.

Tips:

1. Keep your shoulders off the floor and your core engaged throughout the exercise to maximize effectiveness.

2. Focus on using your oblique muscles to reach towards your heels rather than using your arms.

3. Perform the movement slowly and with control to maintain proper form and maximize muscle engagement.

Active Muscles:
Primary: Abdominals (rectus abdominis), Obliques (external and internal obliques)
Secondary: Hip Flexors (iliopsoas)

Equipment:
None

15. Alternate Leg Pull

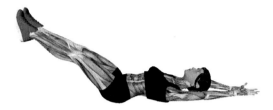

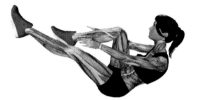

Instructions:
1. Lie on your back with your legs extended straight at 45 degrees off the floor and your arms extended overhead in line with your torso.
2. Lift your shoulders off the mat, engage your core, and simultaneously bring your right knee towards your chest while swinging both arms in an arc motion until parallel to the floor.
3. Straighten your right leg and lower your arms and shoulders back to the starting position.
4. Repeat the movement with your left leg. Continue alternating sides in this manner.

Tips:
1. Keep your core engaged throughout the exercise to maximize muscle activation and protect your lower back.
2. Perform the movement slowly and with control to avoid using momentum and ensure proper form.
3. Breathe steadily, exhale while crunching and bringing your leg towards your chest, and inhale as you lower back down.

Active Muscles:
Primary: Abdominals (rectus abdominis), Hip Flexors (iliopsoas)

Secondary: Quadriceps (quadriceps femoris)

Equipment: None

16. Alternate Leg Raise From Reverse Plank Position

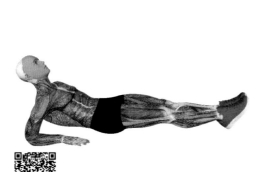

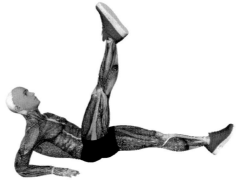

Instructions:

1. Lie down on your hips with your arms resting on the floor by your side and your legs extended forward.

2. Raise your upper back, bring your elbows under the shoulders, and bear weight on your forearms with your palms down.

3. Alternately raise and lower your legs to your maximum range while keeping them straight.

Tips:

1. Focus on maintaining a straight line with your body, avoiding any sagging or arching of the back.

2. Perform the movement slowly and with control to maximize muscle activation and prevent injury.

3. Breathe steadily, exhaling as you lift your leg and inhaling as you lower it back down.

Active Muscles:
Primary: Hip Flexors (iliopsoas), Abdominals (rectus abdominis)
Secondary: Quadriceps (quadriceps femoris)

Equipment:
None

17. Alternate Leg Raise With Head Up

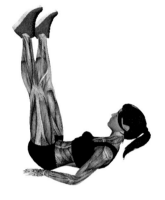 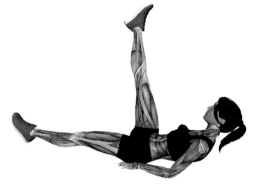

Instructions:

1. Lie down on your back with your arms resting on the floor by your side.

2. Raise your head and upper back off the floor, and lift your legs straight in the air, forming a 90-degree angle with your torso.

3. Lower one of your legs and bring it back just before touching the floor.

4. Do the same with your other leg, and repeat.

Tips:

1. Keep your core engaged throughout the exercise to maintain stability and protect your lower back.

2. Perform the movement slowly and with control to maximize muscle activation and prevent injury.

3. Maintain a steady breathing pattern, exhaling as you lift your leg and inhaling as you lower it back down.

Active Muscles:
Primary: Hip Flexors (iliopsoas), Abdominals (rectus abdominis)
Secondary: Quadriceps (quadriceps femoris)

Equipment:
None

18. Alternate Leg Raise

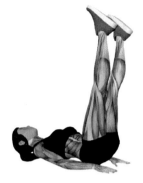

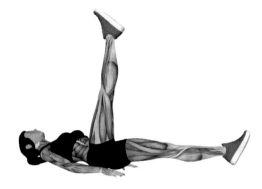

Instructions:

1. Lie down on your back with your arms resting on the floor by your side.
2. Raise your head and upper back off the floor, and lift your legs straight in the air, making a 90-degree angle with your torso.
3. Lower one of your legs and bring it back just before touching the floor.
4. Do the same with your other leg, and repeat.

Tips:

1. Keep your core engaged throughout the exercise to maintain stability and protect your lower back.
2. Perform the movement slowly and with control to maximize muscle activation and prevent injury.
3. Maintain a steady breathing pattern, exhaling as you lift your leg and inhaling as you lower it back down.

Active Muscles:
Primary: Hip Flexors (iliopsoas), Abdominals (rectus abdominis)
Secondary: Quadriceps (quadriceps femoris)

Equipment:
None

19. Alternate Lying Floor Leg Raise

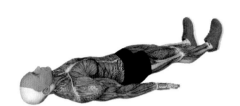
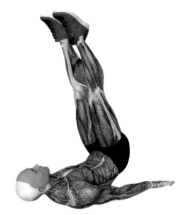

Instructions:

1. Lie on your back with your legs extended straight and your arms resting by your sides.

2. Lift both legs, straight towards the ceiling until they go past your hips.

3. Lower your legs halfway down, then lift them back up towards the ceiling.

4. Lower your legs back down to the initial position. Repeat the movement.

Tips:

1. Focus on keeping your upper back pressed into the mat to avoid arching and straining your spine.

2. Use your breath to guide the movement: inhale as you lift your legs and exhale as you lower them.

3. Engage your thigh muscles to assist with the lift and ensure proper form.

Active Muscles:
Primary: Hip Flexors (iliopsoas), Abdominals (rectus abdominis)
Secondary: Quadriceps (quadriceps femoris)

Equipment:
None

20. Alternate Oblique Crunch

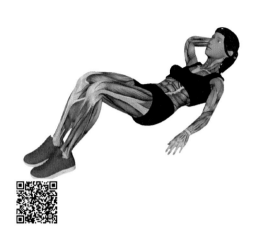

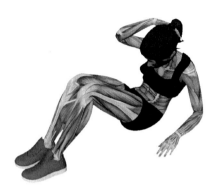

Instructions:

1. Lie down on your back and fold your knees while keeping your feet on the floor.

2. Place your right hand behind your head and your left hand on the floor for support.

3. Raise and twist your chest to your left and bring your right elbow towards the left knee.

4. Return to the starting position and repeat, alternating sides.

Tips:

1. Focus on using your oblique muscles to twist your torso rather than pulling on your neck with your hands.

2. Keep your movements slow and controlled to maximize muscle activation and prevent injury.

3. Ensure your lower back remains pressed into the mat to protect your spine.

Active Muscles:
Primary: Obliques (external and internal obliques)
Secondary: Abdominals (rectus abdominis)
Equipment:
None

21. Alternate Single Leg Raises Plank

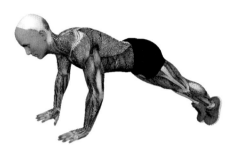 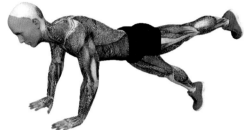

Instructions:

1. Start in a plank position with your hands directly under your shoulders and your body forming a straight line from head to heels.

2. Lift your right leg off the floor, extending it straight back while maintaining the plank position. Hold briefly.

3. Lower your right leg back to the starting position.

4. Lift your left leg off the floor, extending it straight back. Hold briefly before lowering it back to the starting position. Continue alternating sides.

Tips:

1. Keep your core engaged throughout the exercise to maintain stability and prevent your hips from sagging.

2. Perform the movement slowly and with control to maximize muscle activation and prevent injury.

3. Maintain a straight line from head to heels, avoiding any arching or rounding of your back.

Active Muscles:
Primary: Abdominals (rectus abdominis)
Secondary: Glutes (gluteus maximus)

Equipment:
None

22. Alternate Toe Tap Leg Lift

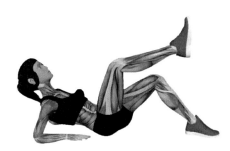
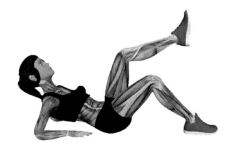

Instructions:
1. Lie down on your back with your knees bent and feet on the floor.
2. Raise your torso off the floor by placing your elbows on the floor and raise one of your knees toward the chest while keeping your knee bent.
3. Lower your foot back to the floor while raising your other knee towards your chest.
4. Keep repeating by alternately moving your knees towards and away from the chest.

Tips:
1. Keep your core engaged throughout the exercise to maintain stability and protect your lower back.
2. Perform the movement slowly and with control to maximize muscle activation and prevent injury.
3. Focus on maintaining the bend in your knees and tapping the floor lightly to ensure proper form.

Active Muscles:
Primary: Hip Flexors (iliopsoas), Abdominals (rectus abdominis)
Secondary: Quadriceps (quadriceps femoris)

Equipment:
None

23. Alternating Leg Lifts

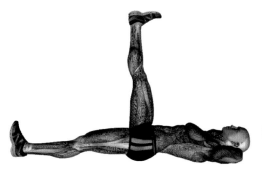
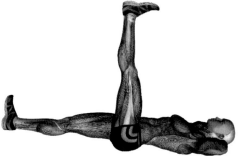

Instructions:
1. Lie down on your back with your legs straight and hands behind your head.

2. Raise one of your legs straight towards the ceiling without bending your knee.

3. Slowly lower your leg back towards the floor and raise the other leg simultaneously.

Tips:
1. Keep your lower back pressed into the floor to maintain proper alignment and avoid strain.

2. Use a controlled breathing pattern: inhale as you lift your leg and exhale as you lower it.

3. Engage your thigh muscles to assist with the lift and maintain straight legs throughout the movement.

Active Muscles:
Primary: Abdominals (rectus abdominis), Hip Flexors (iliopsoas), Quadriceps (quadriceps femoris)
Secondary: Lower Back (erector spinae)

Equipment:
None

24. Alternating Plank Lunge

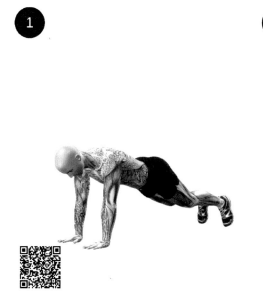

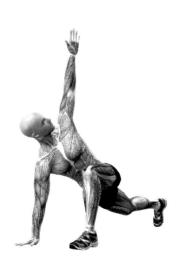

Instructions:

1. Start in a plank position with your hands directly under your shoulders and your body forming a straight line from head to heels.

2. Step your right foot forward outside your right hand, bringing your body into a low lunge position.

3. Lift your left arm, rotate your torso upwards, and lift your arm straight to the ceiling.

4. Return to the starting position and repeat with alternating sides.

Tips:

1. Keep your core engaged throughout the exercise to maintain stability and proper alignment.

2. Ensure your front knee is aligned with your ankle and does not extend past your toes to avoid strain on your knee joint.

3. Perform the movement slowly and with control to maximize muscle activation and prevent injury.

Active Muscles:
Primary: Abdominals (rectus abdominis), Obliques (external and internal obliques), Quadriceps (quadriceps femoris)

Secondary: Hip Flexors (iliopsoas), Triceps (triceps brachii)

Equipment:
None

25. Alternating Toe Tap

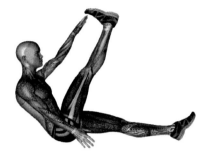

Instructions:

1. Lie on your back with your legs extended straight on the floor and your arms resting by your sides.
2. Simultaneously lift your right leg and left arm towards the ceiling, reaching to touch your toe with your hand.
3. Lower your right leg and left arm back to the starting position.
4. Repeat the movement with your left leg and right arm, lifting them towards the ceiling and trying to touch your toe with your hand. Continue alternating sides.

Tips:

1. Engage your core throughout the exercise to maintain stability and protect your lower back.
2. Perform the movement slowly and with control to maximize muscle activation and prevent injury.
3. Keep your legs straight and avoid bending your knees to ensure proper form.

Active Muscles:
Primary: Abdominals (rectus abdominis), Hip Flexors (iliopsoas)

Secondary: Quadriceps (quadriceps femoris)
Equipment:
None

26. Arm Rotation Knee Lift

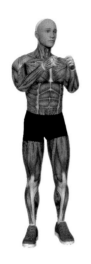

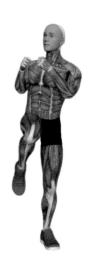

Instructions:

1. Stand tall with your back straight and feet shoulder-width apart.

2. Fold your arms at your sides and make fists with your hands near your chest.

3. Raise your right knee while rotating your torso to the left side and back to the right side.

4. Return to the initial position and repeat by raising your other knee.

Tips:

1. Focus on lifting your knee high to engage your abdominals fully.

2. Use your oblique muscles to initiate the twist, enhancing the rotational movement.

3. Maintain an even pace to ensure both sides of your body work evenly.

Active Muscles:
Primary: Abdominals (rectus abdominis), Hip Flexors (iliopsoas), Obliques (external and internal obliques)

Secondary: Quadriceps (quadriceps femoris), Shoulders (deltoids)
Equipment:
None

27. Assisted Sit-Up

 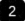

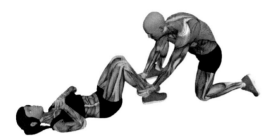 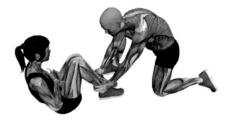

Instructions:

1. Lie on your back on the floor, with your knees bent and feet flat on the floor, close together. Have your partner hold your feet, holding them securely for stability.

2. Cross your arms over your chest or place your hands behind your head.

3. Engage your core and lift your upper body towards your knees.

4. Slowly lower your upper body back to the starting position with control. Repeat the movement for the desired number of repetitions.

Tips:

1. Exhale as you lift your upper body towards your knees and inhale as you lower it back down.

2. Perform the exercise slowly and with control to maximize muscle engagement and effectiveness.

3. If you don't have a partner available, you can place your toes touching the wall in the corner for assistance.

Active Muscles:
Primary: Abdominals (Rectus Abdominis)

Secondary: Obliques (external and internal obliques), Hip Flexors (Iliopsoas)
Equipment:
None

28. Ball Sit-Up

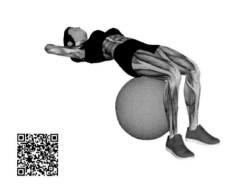

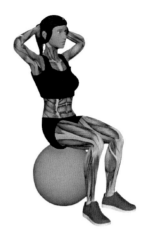

Instructions:

1. Sit on an exercise ball with your feet flat on the floor and knees bent at a 90-degree angle.

2. Lean back, rolling the ball under your lower back, and place your hands behind your head.

3. Engage your core and lift your upper body upwards until vertical to the floor.

4. Lower your upper body back to the starting position, and repeat.

Tips:

1. Keep your core engaged throughout the exercise to maintain stability and proper form.

2. Avoid pulling on your neck with your hands to prevent strain; use your core muscles to lift your body.

3. Perform the movement slowly and with control to maximize muscle activation and prevent injury.

Active Muscles:
Primary: Abdominals (rectus abdominis)
Secondary: Hip Flexors (iliopsoas)

Equipment:
Exercise Ball

29. Bench Decline Ab Sit-Up

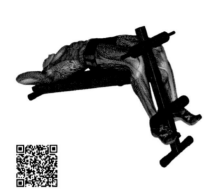

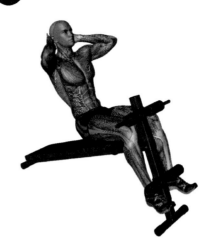

Instructions:

1. Lie on a decline bench with your feet secured under the foot pads.

2. Place your hands behind your head or cross them over your chest.

3. Engage your core and lift your upper body towards your knees until your torso is bent at 90 degrees.

4. Lower your upper body back to the starting position and repeat.

Tips:

1. Ensure your feet are firmly placed under the foot pads for proper support.

2. Focus on squeezing your abdominal muscles at the top of the crunches to enhance muscle engagement.

3. Breathe out as you lift your body and breathe in as you lower it to maintain a steady rhythm and maximize oxygen flow.

Active Muscles:
Primary: Abdominals (rectus abdominis)
Secondary: Hip Flexors (iliopsoas)

Equipment:
Decline Bench

30. Bench Reverse Plank Hold

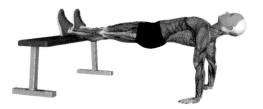 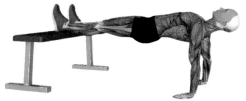

Instructions:
1. Place your feet on a bench with your legs extended, your hands on the floor directly under your shoulders, and your arms straight.
2. Lift your hips straight until your torso comes parallel to the floor.
3. Hold this position, keeping your core engaged and maintaining a straight line from head to heels.
4. Maintain the hold for the designated period, focusing on stability and muscle engagement.

Tips:
1. Engage your core, lower back, and glutes to maintain a straight and stable torso throughout the hold.
2. Keep your elbows slightly bent to avoid locking your joints and ensure muscle engagement.
3. Breathe steadily and avoid holding your breath to maintain control and endurance during the hold.

Active Muscles:
Primary: Abdominals (rectus abdominis), Obliques (external and internal obliques)

Secondary: Lower Back (Erector Spinae), Quadriceps (quadriceps femoris), Shoulders (deltoids)
Equipment:
Bench

31. Bench Knee Tucks

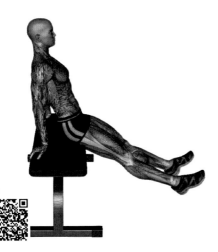
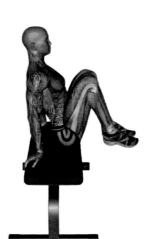

Instructions:

1. Sit on the edge of a bench with your hands holding the bench beside your hips for support.

2. Lean back slightly and lift your feet off the floor with your legs extended straight out.

3. Pull your knees towards your chest, tucking them in while engaging your core.

4. Extend your legs back to the starting position and repeat.

Tips:

1. Keep your core engaged throughout the exercise to maintain stability and proper form.

2. Avoid using momentum; focus on using your abdominal muscles to pull your knees in.

3. Breathe steadily, exhaling as you tuck your knees in and inhaling as you extend your legs out.

Active Muscles:
Primary: Abdominals (rectus abdominis)
Secondary: Hip Flexors (iliopsoas)

Equipment:
Bench

32. Bent Knee Lying Twist (On Stability Ball)

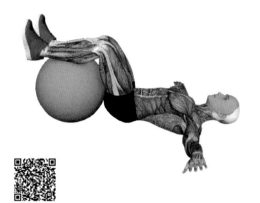 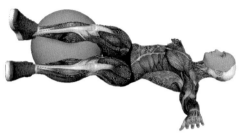

Instructions:

1. Lie on the floor with your arms extended out to the sides to form a T shape.

2. Place your bent legs on top of an exercise ball.

3. Lower your bent knees to one side, keeping your torso and arms flat on the floor.

4. Then, bring your knees back to the center and lower them to the opposite side. Repeat the movement for the desired number of repetitions.

Tips:

1. Keep your shoulders flat on the floor to maximize the stretch in your spine and obliques.

2. Move slowly and with control to avoid straining your back.

3. Breathe deeply and steadily, exhaling as you lower your knees to the side and inhaling as you bring them back to the center.

Active Muscles:
Primary: Obliques (external and internal obliques), Abdominals (rectus abdominis)
Secondary: Lower Back (erector spinae)

Equipment:
Exercise Ball

33. Bent Knee Lying Twist

1

2

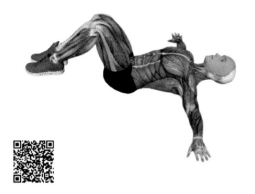
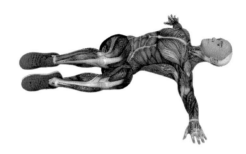

Instructions:
1. Lie on your back with your arms extended out to the sides, forming a T shape.

2. Bend your knees and lift your feet off the floor, bringing your upper legs vertically to the floor.

3. Lower your bent knees to one side, keeping your torso and arms flat on the floor.

4. Then, bring your knees back to the center and lower them to the opposite side. Repeat the movement for the desired number of repetitions.

Tips:
1. Keep your shoulders flat on the floor to maximize the stretch in your spine and obliques.

2. Move slowly and with control to avoid straining your back.

3. Breathe deeply and steadily, exhaling as you lower your knees to the side and inhaling as you bring them back to the center.

Active Muscles:
Primary: Obliques (external and internal obliques), Abdominals (rectus abdominis)
Secondary: Lower Back (erector spinae)

Equipment:
None

34. Bicycle Air Legs

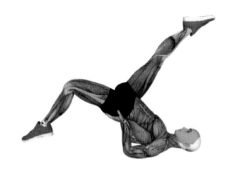

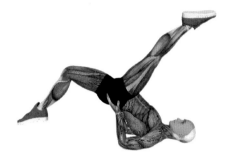

Instructions:

1. Lie on your back and lift your hips off the floor, supporting them with your hands while keeping your elbows on the floor.

2. Perform a bicycle motion with your legs by extending your right leg straight forward while bending your left knee towards the floor.

3. Switch legs by extending your left leg straight forward and bending your right knee towards the floor, continuing the bicycle motion.

4. Maintain a controlled and steady pace throughout the exercise.

Tips:

1. Ensure your hands firmly support your lower back to maintain proper alignment and stability.

2. Focus on engaging your core muscles to control the move-ment of your legs and prevent lower back strain.

3. Ensure your movements are smooth and controlled to maximize muscle activation and prevent injury.

Active Muscles:
Primary: Abdominals (rectus abdominis), Hip Flexors (iliopsoas)
Secondary: Quadriceps (quadriceps femoris), Hamstrings (biceps femoris, semitendinosus, semimembranosus)
Equipment:
None

35. Bicycle Twisting Crunch

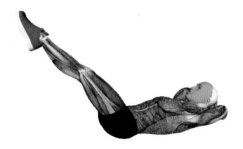
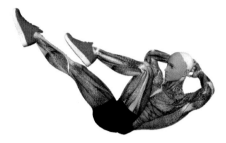

Instructions:

1. Lie on your back with your hands behind your head and your legs raised at 45 degrees off the floor, keeping them straight.

2. Bring your right knee towards your chest while twisting your torso, bringing your left elbow towards your right knee.

3. Alternate sides, bringing your left knee towards your chest and your right elbow towards your left knee, continuing in a controlled, bicycle-like motion.

Tips:

1. Focus on using your abdominal muscles to twist rather than your neck or shoulders.

4. Ensure your lower back stays pressed against the floor throughout the exercise to prevent strain.

5. Avoid pulling on your neck with your hands; use your core muscles to lift and twist your torso.

Active Muscles:
Primary: Abdominals (rectus abdominis), Obliques (external and internal obliques)
Secondary: Hip Flexors (iliopsoas), Quadriceps (quadriceps femoris)

Equipment:
None

36. Bicycles Crunches

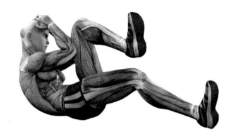

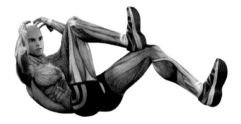

Instructions:

1. Lie on your back with your hands behind your head and your legs lifted off the floor.

2. Bring your right knee towards your chest while extending your left leg out.

3. Simultaneously twist your torso, bringing your left elbow towards your right knee.

4. Alternate sides, bringing your left knee towards your chest and your right elbow towards your left knee, continuing in a controlled, bicycle-like motion.

Tips:

1. Focus on using your abdominal muscles to perform the twist, rather than your neck or shoulders.

2. Ensure your lower back stays pressed against the floor throughout the exercise to prevent strain.

3. Keep your elbows wide and avoid pulling on your head to prevent neck strain.

Active Muscles:
Primary: Abdominals (rectus abdominis), Obliques (external and internal obliques)

Secondary: Hip Flexors (iliopsoas), Quadriceps (quadriceps femoris)
Equipment:
None

37. Bicycles

1

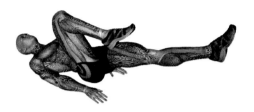

2

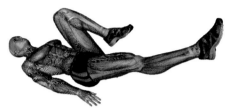

Instructions:
1. Lie on your back with your legs bent and lifted off the floor, and both arms straight to the floor.
2. Bring your right knee towards your chest while straightening your left leg towards the floor without letting it touch the floor.
3. Alternate sides by bringing your left knee towards your chest and straightening your right leg towards the floor, continuing in a controlled, bicycle-like motion.

Tips:
1. Focus on using your abdominal muscles to control the movement of your legs.
2. Ensure your lower back stays pressed against the floor throughout the exercise to prevent strain.
3. Keep your movements slow and controlled to maximize muscle activation and avoid injury.

Active Muscles:
Primary: Abdominals (rectus abdominis), Hip Flexors (iliopsoas)
Secondary: Quadriceps (quadriceps femoris)

Equipment:
None

38. Body Saw Plank

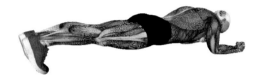

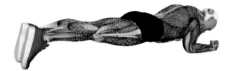

Instructions:

1. Start in a forearm plank position, with your elbows directly under your shoulders and your body forming a straight line from head to heels.
2. Rock your body back by pushing through your forearms, moving your shoulders behind your elbows level.
3. Rock your body forward by pulling with your forearms, moving your shoulders in front of your elbows level.
4. Repeat this controlled forward and backward motion.

Tips:

1. Focus on keeping your body straight from head to heels to maintain proper form.
2. Ensure your movements are slow and deliberate to enhance control and muscle engagement.
3. Breathe steadily, exhaling as you rock forward and inhaling as you rock back.

Active Muscles:
Primary: Core Muscles (rectus abdominis, obliques), Shoulders (deltoids)

Secondary: Lower Back (erector spinae), Glutes (gluteus maximus), Hip Flexors (iliopsoas)
Equipment:
None

39. Bottoms-Up Half Rep

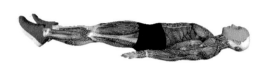

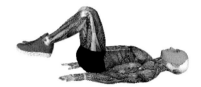

Instructions:
1. Lie on your back with your legs extended just off the floor and your arms resting on the floor by your sides.
2. Bend your knees towards your chest, stopping when your upper legs are vertical to the floor.
3. Lower your legs back down without letting them touch the floor.
4. Repeat the movement for the desired number of repetitions.

Tips:
1. Keep your core engaged throughout the exercise to maintain stability and support your lower back.
2. Perform the movement slowly and with control to maximize muscle activation and prevent injury.
3. Focus on using your lower abdominal muscles to lift and lower your legs.

Active Muscles:
Primary: Abdominals (Rectus Abdominis)
Secondary: Hip Flexors (Iliopsoas)

Equipment:
None

40. Brazilian Crunches

 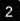

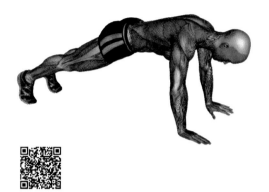 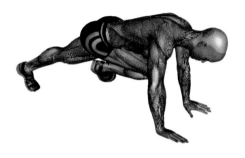

Instructions:

1. Begin in a plank position on your toes and hands, arms straight in line with shoulders, with your body in a straight line from head to heels.

2. Bend your right knee and bring it towards your left elbow while lightly rotating your hips. Return your leg to the starting position.

3. Repeat the movement on the opposite side, bending your left knee and bringing it towards your right elbow while lightly rotating your hips. Continue alternating sides for the desired number of repetitions.

Tips:

1. Keep your movements controlled to ensure each repetition is deliberate and effective.

2. Maintain a steady breathing pattern, exhaling as you bring your knee towards your elbow and inhaling as you return to the plank.

3. Focus on maintaining proper plank form and keeping your body straight from head to heels.

Active Muscles:
Primary: Abdominals (Rectus Abdominis, Obliques)

Secondary: Shoulders (Deltoids), Hip Flexors (Iliopsoas)
Equipment:
None

41. Bridge - Mountain Climber (Cross Body)

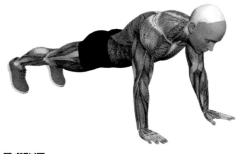 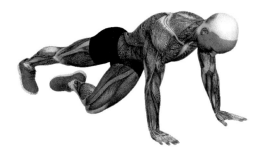

Instructions:

1. Begin in a plank position on your toes and hands, with your body in a straight line from head to heels.

2. Bend your right knee and bring it towards your left elbow while lightly rotating your hips. Stop when your knee passes the elbow.

3. Return to the starting plank position, then repeat the movement on the opposite side.

4. Continue alternating sides for the desired number of repetitions.

Tips:

1. Ensure you keep your movement smooth and controlled to maintain form and avoid injury.

2. Maintain a steady breathing pattern, exhaling as you bring your knee towards your elbow and inhaling as you return to the plank position.

3. Keep your shoulders stable and your core engaged throughout the exercise to enhance effectiveness.

Active Muscles:
Primary: Abdominals (Rectus Abdominis, Obliques)

Secondary: Shoulders (Deltoids), Hip Flexors (Iliopsoas)
Equipment:
None

42. Captain's Chair Leg Raise

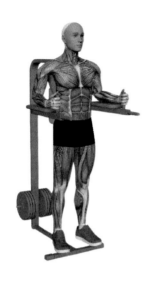

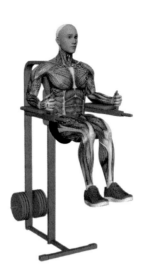

Instructions:

1. Stand on the platform of the captain's chair and place your forearms on the arm pads, gripping the handles for stability. Allow your legs to hang straight down.

2. Engage your core and keep your back pressed against the back pad.

3. Raise your legs, knees first, up in front of you until your thighs are parallel to the floor and your feet are slightly forward.

4. Slowly lower your knees back to the starting position with control. Repeat for the desired number of repetitions.

Tips:

1. Keep your back pressed against the back pad to prevent swinging and maintain proper form.

2. Avoid using momentum; the movement should be controlled and deliberate.

3. Exhale as you raise your legs and inhale as you lower them back down.

Active Muscles:
Primary: Abdominals (Rectus Abdominis)

Secondary: Hip Flexors (Iliopsoas), Quadriceps (Quadriceps Femoris)
Equipment:
Captain's Chair

43. Captain's Chair Straight Leg Raise

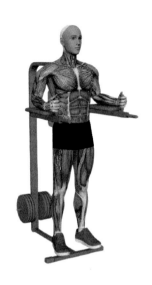

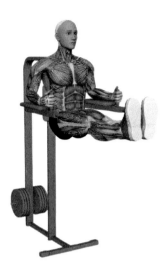

Instructions:

1. Stand on the platform of the captain's chair and place your forearms on the arm pads, gripping the handles for stability. Allow your legs to hang straight down.

2. Engage your core and keep your back pressed against the back pad.

3. Raise your legs straight up in front of you until they are parallel to the floor, keeping them as straight as possible.

4. Slowly lower your legs back to the starting position with control. Repeat for the desired number of repetitions.

Tips:

1. Keep your back pressed against the back pad to prevent swinging and maintain proper form.

2. Avoid using momentum; the movement should be controlled and deliberate.

3. Exhale as you raise your legs and inhale as you lower them back down.

Active Muscles:
Primary: Abdominals (Rectus Abdominis)

Secondary: Hip Flexors (Iliopsoas), Quadriceps (Quadriceps Femoris)
Equipment:
Captain's Chair

44. Chest Lift With Rotation

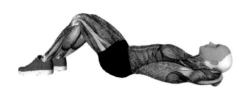

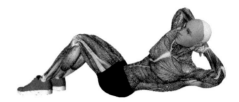

Instructions:

1. Begin by lying on your back with your knees bent and feet flat on the floor. Place your hands behind your head with your elbows wide.

2. Engage your core and lift your upper body slightly into a crunch position, holding the contraction at the top for a second.

3. While holding the crunch, rotate your torso to the right and return to the center.

4. Lower your upper body back to the floor, then repeat the movement, rotating to the left. Continue alternating sides for the desired number of repetitions.

Tips:

1. Avoid pulling on your neck with your hands; use your abdominal muscles to lift and rotate your torso.

2. Keep your elbows wide to ensure you use your core muscles rather than your arms.

3. Ensure your lower back remains pressed against the floor throughout the exercise.

Active Muscles:
Primary: Rectus Abdominis (Abdominals), Obliques (Sides of the abdomen)

Secondary: Lower Back (erector spinae)
Equipment:
None

45. Crab Pose

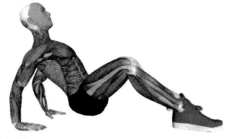

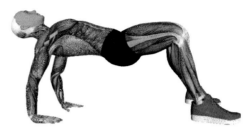

Instructions:

1. Begin by sitting on the floor with your legs bent, feet flat on the floor, and hands placed behind you with your fingers pointing away from your body.

2. Engage your core and press through your palms and feet to lift your hips off the floor, creating a tabletop position with your body.

3. Hold this position, ensuring your hips are lifted high, and your torso is parallel to the floor while keeping your head in line with your spine.

4. After holding the position for the desired duration, slowly lower your hips back to the floor and return to the starting position.

Tips:

1. Focus on pressing through your palms and feet to lift your hips as high as possible, creating a straight line from your shoulders to your knees.

2. To prevent discomfort during the exercise, use a mat or soft surface to support your hands and feet.

3. Ensure your shoulders remain down and away from your ears to avoid unnecessary strain.

Active Muscles:
Primary: Core Muscles (Rectus Abdominis, Obliques), Hamstrings (Biceps Femoris)

Secondary: Triceps (Triceps Brachii), Shoulders (Deltoids)
Equipment:
None

The Ultimate Exercise Guide: Abdominals Edition - 1st Edition

46. Crab Twist Toe Touch

1

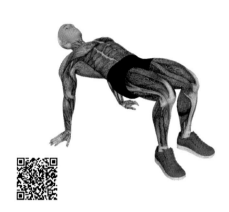

2

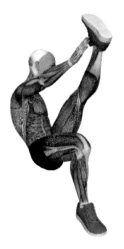

Instructions:

1. Begin by sitting on the floor with your legs bent, feet flat on the floor, and hands placed behind you with your fingers pointing away from your body.

2. Engage your glutes and press through your palms and feet to lift your hips off the floor, creating a tabletop position with your body.

3. Simultaneously lift your right hand and left foot off the floor and twist your torso to reach your right hand towards your left foot, attempting to touch your left toe.

4. Return your hand and leg to the floor and repeat the movement on the opposite side. Continue alternating sides for the desired number of repetitions.

Tips:

1. Perform the twist with control to maximize muscle activation and prevent injury.

2. Ensure your shoulders remain down and away from your ears to avoid unnecessary strain.

3. Breathe steadily throughout the exercise, exhaling as you twist and reach towards your toe and inhaling as you return to the starting position.

Active Muscles:
Primary: Core Muscles (Rectus Abdominis, Obliques), Hamstrings (Biceps Femoris)

Secondary: Triceps (Triceps Brachii), Shoulders (Deltoids)
Equipment:
None

47. Criss Cross Leg Raises

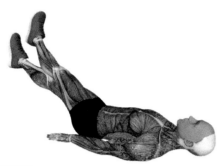

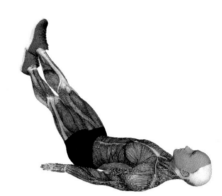

Instructions:

1. Begin by lying flat on your back with your legs extended straight out and your arms resting by your sides or under your lower back for support. Engage your core and lift both legs slightly off the floor.

2. Start crisscrossing your legs in a scissor motion, crossing your right leg over your left and then your left leg over your right.

3. Gradually move your legs upward while continuing to crisscross until they form a 45-degree angle with your torso. Then, lower them back down to just above the floor, maintaining the crisscross motion throughout.

4. Repeat the movement for the desired number of repetitions.

Tips:

1. Keep your core engaged throughout the exercise to maintain stability and support your lower back.

2. Focus on using your leg muscles to control the movement, keeping your legs straight and performing the crisscross motion smoothly.

3. Ensure your lower back remains pressed into the floor to avoid unnecessary strain.

Active Muscles:
Primary: Core (Rectus Abdominis, Obliques), Hip Flexors (Iliopsoas)

Secondary: Quadriceps (Quadriceps Femoris)
Equipment:
None

The Ultimate Exercise Guide: Abdominals Edition - 1st Edition

48. Crunch (Arms Straight)

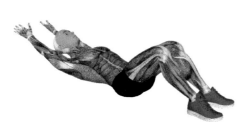

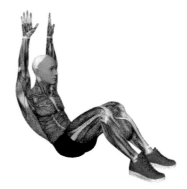

Instructions:

1. Begin by lying flat on your back with your knees bent and your feet flat on the floor, hip-width apart.

2. Extend your arms straight above your head, keeping them aligned with your ears.

3. Engage your core and lift your back off the floor, reaching your arms straight up towards the ceiling.

4. Lower your back to the floor with control, keeping your arms extended. Repeat the movement for the desired number of repetitions.

Tips:

1. Avoid using your neck or momentum to lift your shoulders; focus on using your abdominal muscles.

2. Use a mat or soft surface to support your back and prevent discomfort during the exercise.

3. Breathe steadily throughout the exercise, exhaling as you lift your shoulders and inhaling as you lower them.

Active Muscles:
Primary: Abdominals (Rectus Abdominis)
Secondary: Obliques (external and internal obliques)

Equipment:
None

49. Crunch (Hands Overhead)

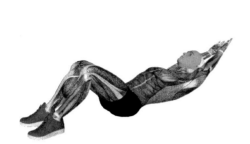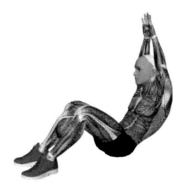

Instructions:

1. Begin by lying flat on your back with your knees bent and your feet flat on the floor, hip-width apart.

2. Extend your arms straight overhead with hands close together, keeping them in line with your ears.

3. Engage your core and lift your back off the floor, reaching your hands straight up towards the ceiling.

4. Lower your back to the floor with control, keeping your arms extended. Repeat the movement for the desired number of repetitions.

Tips:

1. Avoid using your neck or momentum to lift your shoulders; focus on using your abdominal muscles.

2. Perform the movement with control to maximize muscle activation and prevent injury.

3. Breathe steadily throughout the exercise, exhaling as you lift your shoulders and inhaling as you lower them.

Active Muscles:
Primary: Abdominals (Rectus Abdominis)

Secondary: Obliques (external and internal obliques)
Equipment:
None

50. Crunch With Legs On Stability Ball

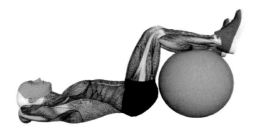 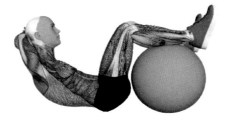

Instructions:

1. Begin by lying flat on your back with your knees bent at a 90-degree angle and your lower legs resting on a stability ball.

2. Place your hands behind your head with your elbows pointing out to the sides.

3. Lift your back off the floor, curling your upper body towards your knees while keeping your legs stable on the ball.

4. Lower your back to the floor with control, maintaining your legs' position on the ball. Repeat the movement for the desired number of repetitions.

Tips:

1. Keep your core engaged throughout the exercise to maintain stability and support your lower back.

2. Avoid pulling on your neck with your hands; focus on using your abdominal muscles to lift your shoulders.

3. Breathe steadily throughout the exercise, exhaling as you lift your shoulders and inhaling as you lower them.

Active Muscles:
Primary: Abdominals (Rectus Abdominis)

Secondary: Obliques (external and internal obliques)
Equipment:
Stability/Exercise Ball

51. Crunch (On BOSU Ball)

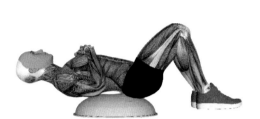
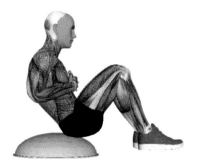

Instructions:

1. Begin by sitting on a BOSU ball with your feet flat on the floor and your knees bent.

2. Lean back to position your lower back against the BOSU ball, ensuring your upper body is supported. Place your hands behind your head with your elbows pointing out to the sides, or on your chest.

3. Engage your core and lift your back upwards, curling your upper body towards your knees.

4. Lower your back down with control, maintaining your core engagement. Repeat the movement for the desired number of repetitions.

Tips:

1. Avoid pulling on your neck with your hands; focus on using your abdominal muscles to lift your shoulders.

2. Use a mat or soft surface under the BOSU ball if need-ed for additional stability and comfort.

3. Breathe steadily throughout the exercise, exhaling as you lift your shoulders and inhaling as you lower them.

Active Muscles:
Primary: Abdominals (Rectus Abdominis)

Secondary: Obliques (external and internal obliques)
Equipment:
BOSU

52. Crunch (On Stability Ball)

 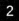

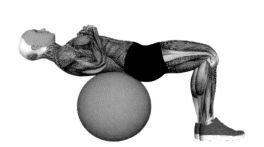 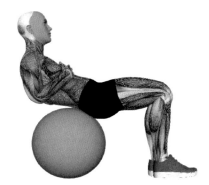

Instructions:

1. Begin by sitting on a stability ball with your feet flat on the floor and your knees bent at a 90-degree angle.

2. Walk your feet forward and lean back to position your lower back on the stability ball. Place your hands behind your head with your elbows pointing out to the sides, or on your chest.

3. Engage your core and lift your back upwards, curling your upper body towards your knees.

4. Lower your upper back down with control, maintaining your core engagement. Repeat the movement for the desired number of repetitions.

Tips:

1. Avoid pulling on your neck with your hands; focus on using your abdominal muscles to lift your back.

2. Ensure your lower back remains in contact with the stability ball to avoid unnecessary strain.

3. Breathe steadily throughout the exercise, exhaling as you lift your shoulders and inhaling as you lower them.

Active Muscles:
Primary: Abdominals (Rectus Abdominis)

Secondary: Obliques (external and internal obliques)
Equipment:
Stability/Exercise Ball

53. Crunch (Straight Leg Up)

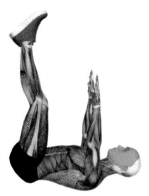
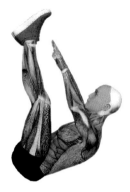

Instructions:
1. Begin by lying flat on your back with your legs extended straight up towards the ceiling. Keep your feet together and your arms extended straight above your chest.

2. Engage your core and lift your back off the floor, reaching your arms towards your toes.

3. Hold the crunch position briefly, squeezing your abdominal muscles at the top.

4. Lower your back to the floor with control, keeping your legs extended upward. Repeat the movement for the desired number of repetitions.

Tips:
1. Avoid using your neck or momentum to lift your shoulders; focus on using your abdominal muscles.

2. Use a mat or soft surface to support your back and prevent discomfort during the exercise.

3. Breathe steadily throughout the exercise, exhaling as you lift your shoulders and inhaling as you lower them.

Active Muscles:
Primary: Abdominals (Rectus Abdominis)
Secondary: Hip Flexors (Iliopsoas)

Equipment:
None

54. Crunch Floor

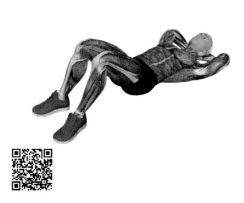
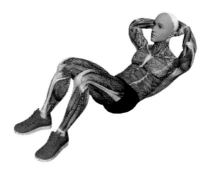

Instructions:

1. Begin by lying flat on your back with your knees bent and your feet flat on the floor, hip-width apart.

2. Place your hands behind your head with your elbows pointing out to the sides.

3. Engage your core and lift your back off the floor, curling your upper body towards your knees.

4. Lower your back to the floor with control, maintaining your core engagement. Repeat the movement for the desired number of repetitions.

Tips:

1. Avoid pulling on your neck with your hands; focus on using your abdominal muscles to lift your shoulders.

2. Perform the movement with control to maximize muscle activation and prevent injury.

3. Breathe steadily throughout the exercise, exhaling as you lift your shoulders and inhaling as you lower them.

Active Muscles:
Primary: Abdominals (Rectus Abdominis)

Secondary: Hip Flexors (Iliopsoas), Obliques (External Obliques, Internal Obliques)
Equipment:
None

55. Crunch Frog On Floor

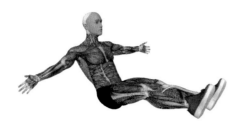
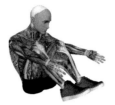

Instructions:
1. Begin seated on the floor, leaning back slightly. Your arms should be extended out to the sides at shoulder level, and your legs should be extended straight and parallel just above the floor.
2. Engage your core to simultaneously bring both knees towards your chest while lightly crunching your upper body towards your knees.
3. As you crunch, bring your arms together towards the sides of your knees.
4. Extend your legs back out and open your arms back to the starting position with control. Repeat the movement for the desired number of repetitions.

Tips:
1. Focus on using your abdominal muscles to lift your legs and upper body, avoiding excessive use of momentum.
2. Ensure your lower back remains stable and avoid arching it during the movement.
3. Breathe steadily throughout the exercise, exhaling as you crunch and inhaling as you extend back out.

Active Muscles:
Primary: Abdominals (Rectus Abdominis), Obliques (External Obliques, Internal Obliques)

Secondary: Hip Flexors (Iliopsoas), Quadriceps (Quadriceps Femoris)
Equipment:
None

56. Crunch Leg Raise

1

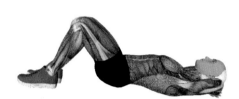

2

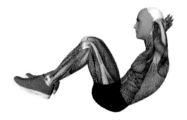

Instructions:
1. Begin by lying flat on your back with your knees bent and your feet just off the floor.

2. Place your hands behind your head with your elbows pointing out to the sides.

3. Engage your core and lift your back off the floor while lifting your legs slightly to bring your knees towards your head.

4. Lower your back to the floor and your legs back to the starting position, keeping your feet just off the floor. Repeat the movement for the desired number of repetitions.

Tips:
1. Avoid using your neck or momentum to lift your shoulders; focus on using your abdominal muscles.

2. Use a mat or soft surface to support your back and prevent discomfort during the exercise.

3. Breathe steadily throughout the exercise, exhaling as you lift your shoulders and knees and inhaling as you lower them.

Active Muscles:
Primary: Abdominals (Rectus Abdominis), Obliques (External Obliques, Internal Obliques)

Secondary: Hip Flexors (Iliopsoas), Quadriceps (Quadriceps Femoris)
Equipment:
None

57. Dead Bug Extended Arms

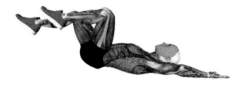
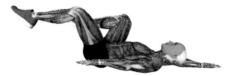

Instructions:

1. Begin by lying flat on your back, right arm extended overhead on the floor in line with your torso and left arm extended by your side. Right knee bent close to your chest, while the left leg is bent and lightly extended away from your hips, keeping both lower legs parallel to the floor.

2. In an arc motion bring your right arm to your side while slowly extending your right leg to pass your hip level and simultaneously bring your left arm in an arc motion extended overhead on the floor in line with your torso and left knee closer to your chest.

3. Repeat the movement with the opposite arm and leg. Continue alternating sides for the desired number of repetitions.

Tips:

1. Breathe steadily throughout the exercise, exhaling as you lower your arm and leg and inhaling as you return to the starting position.

2. Avoid letting your leg touch the floor; keep it just above the floor to maintain tension in your muscles.

3. Use a mat or soft surface to support your back and prevent discomfort during the exercise.

Active Muscles:
Primary: Abdominals (Rectus Abdominis), Obliques (External Obliques, Internal Obliques)

Secondary: Hip Flexors (Iliopsoas), Quadriceps (Quadriceps Femoris)
Equipment:
None

58. Dead Bug

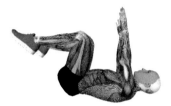
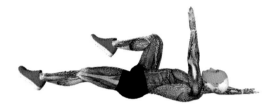

Instructions:
1. Begin by lying flat on your back, arms extended straight up towards the ceiling, legs lifted, and knees bent at a 90-degree angle.

2. Engage your core and slowly lower your right arm and left leg towards the floor, keeping your back flat on the floor and not allowing it to arch.

3. Return your right arm and left leg to the starting position.

4. Repeat the movement with your left arm and right leg. Continue alternating sides for the desired number of repetitions.

Tips:
1. Keep your core engaged throughout the exercise to maintain stability and support your lower back.

2. Avoid letting your leg touch the floor; keep it just above the floor to maintain tension in your muscles.

3. Ensure your lower back remains pressed into the floor to avoid unnecessary strain.

Active Muscles:
Primary: Abdominals (Rectus Abdominis), Obliques (External Obliques, Internal Obliques)

Secondary: Hip Flexors (Iliopsoas), Quadriceps (Quadriceps Femoris)
Equipment:
None

59. Decline Bench Oblique Crunches

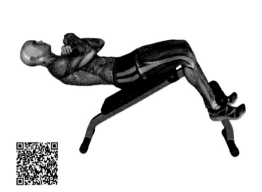
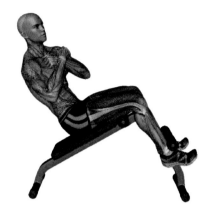

Instructions:

1. Secure your feet at the end of a decline bench, lie back with your knees slightly bent, and cross your hands close to your chest.

2. Engage your core and lift your upper body off the bench while twisting your torso to the right.

3. Squeeze your obliques at the top of the movement, ensuring that the contraction is felt along the side of your abdomen.

4. Slowly lower your upper body back to the starting position and repeat the movement, twisting your torso to the left. Continue alternating sides for the desired number of repetitions.

Tips:

1. Breathe out as you twist and crunch and breathe in as you return to the starting position.

2. Ensure your lower back stays in contact with the bench to support your spine.

3. Keep your feet securely anchored to the bench to stabilize your body throughout the exercise.

Active Muscles:
Primary: Obliques (Internal and External Obliques), Abdominals (Rectus Abdominis)

Secondary: Hip Flexors (Iliopsoas)
Equipment:
Decline Bench

60. Decline Sit-up

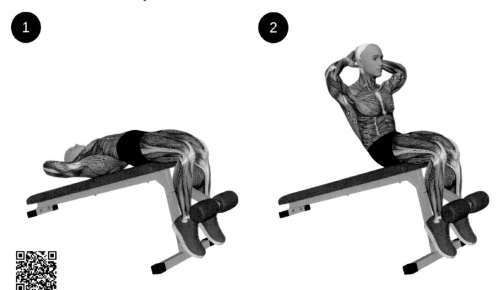

Instructions:

1. Lie on a decline bench with your feet secured under the footpads. Position yourself so that your hips are at the edge of the bench.

2. Place your hands behind your head with your elbows pointing out to the sides.

3. Engage your core and lift your upper body towards your knees until your torso forms a 90-degree angle with your thighs, keeping your back as straight as possible.

4. Lower your upper body back to the starting position with control. Repeat the movement for the desired number of repetitions.

Tips:

1. Keep your core engaged throughout the exercise to maintain stability and support your lower back.

2. Avoid pulling on your neck with your hands; focus on using your abdominal muscles to lift your shoulders.

3. Breathe steadily throughout the exercise, exhaling as you lift your shoulders and inhaling as you lower them.

Active Muscles:
Primary: Abdominals (Rectus Abdominis), Obliques (Internal and External Obliques)

Secondary: Hip Flexors (Iliopsoas)
Equipment:
Decline Bench

61. Decline Bent Leg Reverse Crunch

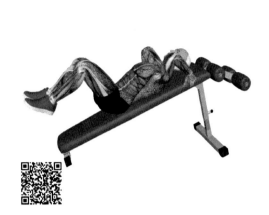

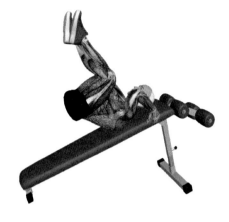

Instructions:

1. Begin by lying on a decline bench with your head at the higher end. Hold the side edges of the bench for stability. Bend your knees at 90 degrees and lift your legs so your thighs are perpendicular to the bench and your lower legs are parallel to the floor.

2. Engage your core and lift your hips off the bench, curling your knees towards your chest while keeping both legs bent.

3. Lower your hips back to the starting position with control, keeping your knees bent at 90 degrees. Repeat the movement for the desired number of repetitions.

Tips:

1. Keep your core engaged throughout the exercise to maintain stability and support your lower back.

2. Avoid using momentum to lift your hips; focus on using your abdominal muscles for the movement.

3. Breathe steadily throughout the exercise, exhaling as you lift your hips and inhaling as you lower them.

Active Muscles:
Primary: Abdominals (Rectus Abdominis)

Secondary: Hip Flexors (Iliopsoas)
Equipment:
Decline Bench

62. Diagonal Chop

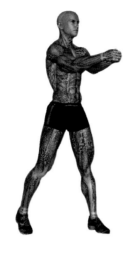

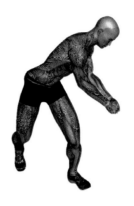

Instructions:
1. Start standing with your feet shoulder-width apart, clasping your hands together and holding them extended opposite your chest.

2. Rotate your torso and bring your hands diagonally across your body towards your left hip, bending your knees slightly as you turn.

3. Keep your arms extended and pivot your right foot as you rotate and return to the starting position in a controlled manner.

4. Repeat the movement for the desired number of repetitions.

Tips:
1. Engage your core throughout the movement to stabilize your spine and enhance power.

2. Pivot your feet during the rotation to ensure a full range of motion and reduce stress on your knees.

3. Focus on exhaling as you chop down and inhaling as you return to the starting position.

Active Muscles:
Primary: Obliques (External Oblique, Internal Oblique)
Secondary: Shoulders (Deltoids)

Equipment:
None

63. Elbow Push Plank Up

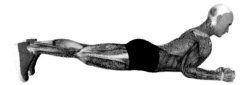

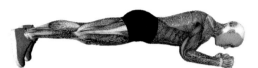

Instructions:

1. Begin in a forearm plank position with your elbows under your shoulders and your body forming an arch line from your head to your heels.

2. Push through your forearms to lift your elbows a few inches off the floor, keeping your fists on the floor.

3. Keep pressing through your forearms to raise your hips off the floor until your torso is straight, maintaining the plank position.

4. Lower your hips back down to the floor, followed by your elbows, returning to the starting position. Repeat for the desired number of repetitions.

Tips:

1. Perform the exercise on a non-slip surface to prevent your forearms from slipping.

2. Ensure your elbows remain under your shoulders to maintain proper form and prevent strain.

3. Move slowly and with control to maximize muscle engagement and prevent injury.

Active Muscles:
Primary: Core muscles (Rectus Abdominis, Obliques)
Secondary: Shoulders (Deltoids), Triceps (Triceps Brachii)

Equipment:
None

64. Exercise Ball Body Saw

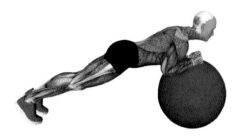
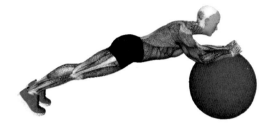

Instructions:

1. Begin in a plank position with your forearms resting on an exercise ball and your body forming a straight line from your head to your heels.

2. Engage your core and slowly roll the ball a few inches away from your body.

3. Reverse the motion by rolling the ball closer to your forearms.

4. Continue the rolling motion for the desired number of repetitions.

Tips:

1. Breathe steadily throughout the exercise, exhaling as you move forward and inhaling as you move back.

2. Avoid allowing your lower back to arch; keep your spine neutral.

3. Use a properly inflated exercise ball to ensure stability and control during the movement.

Active Muscles:
Primary: Core muscles (Rectus Abdominis, Obliques)
Secondary: Shoulders (Deltoids), Triceps (Triceps Brachii)

Equipment:
Exercise Ball

65. Flutter Kicks

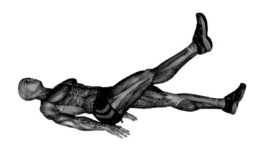

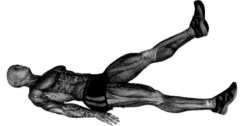

Instructions:

1. Lie on your back with your legs extended and your arms at your sides, palms facing down.

2. Lift your legs off the floor a few inches, keeping them straight and close together.

3. Quickly alternate kicking your legs up and down in a small, controlled motion, engaging your core throughout the movement.

4. Continue the flutter kicks for the desired duration, maintaining a steady and controlled pace.

Tips:

1. Move your legs in a controlled manner to maximize muscle engagement and prevent injury.

2. Focus on steady breathing, exhaling as you kick your legs and inhaling as you maintain the movement.

3. Avoid letting your lower back arch off the floor; keep it pressed down to prevent strain.

Active Muscles:
Primary: Abdominals (Rectus Abdominis)
Secondary: Hip Flexors (Iliopsoas)

Equipment:
None

66. Hanging Knee Raises

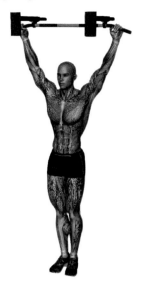

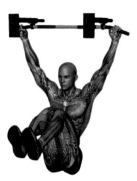

Instructions:

1. Hang from a pull-up bar with your hands shoulder-width apart, palms facing forward or towards each other. Allow your body to hang straight with your feet off the floor.

2. Keeping your legs together, bend your knees and lift them towards your chest.

3. Raise your knees as high as comfortably possible, aiming to bring them towards your chest.

4. Slowly lower your legs back to the starting position with control. Repeat for the desired number of repetitions.

Tips:

1. Avoid swinging your body; use controlled movements to lift and lower your legs.

2. Focus on steady breathing, exhaling as you lift your knees and inhaling as you lower them.

3. Ensure your grip on the bar is secure to prevent slipping.

Active Muscles:
Primary: Abdominals (Rectus Abdominis)
Secondary: Hip Flexors (Iliopsoas)

Equipment:
None

67. Hanging Oblique Crunches

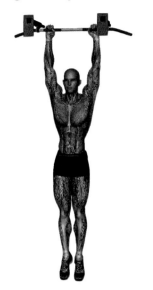

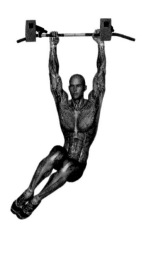

Instructions:

1. Hang from a pull-up bar with your hands shoulder-width apart, palms facing forward or towards each other. Allow your body to hang straight with your feet off the floor.

2. Keeping your legs together, bend your knees and lift them towards your right elbow, twisting your torso to engage your obliques.

3. Raise your knees as high as comfortably possible, aiming to bring them towards your elbow.

4. Slowly lower your legs back to the starting position with control. Repeat the movement, alternating sides for the desired number of repetitions.

Tips:

1. Avoid swinging your body; use controlled movements to lift and lower your legs.

2. Focus on steady breathing, exhaling as you lift your knees and twist and inhaling as you lower them.

3. Ensure your grip on the bar is secure to prevent slipping.

Active Muscles:
Primary: Obliques (External Obliques, Internal Obliques), Abdominals (Rectus Abdominis)

Secondary: Hip Flexors (Iliopsoas)
Equipment:
None

68. High Knee Twist

 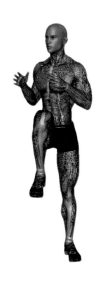

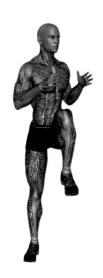

Instructions:
1. Stand with your feet hip-width apart and your arms raised to shoulder height in front of you, palms facing down.

2. Lift your right knee towards your left elbow while simultaneously twisting your torso to the right.

3. Return to the starting position, then lift your left knee towards your right elbow while twisting your torso to the left.

4. Alternate sides in a controlled manner, maintaining a steady rhythm. Repeat for the desired number of repetitions.

Tips:
1. Twist your torso and lift your knee simultaneously to engage your abs and obliques.

2. Move smoothly and with control to avoid straining your back or hips.

3. Ensure your movements are balanced and controlled to prevent injury.

Active Muscles:
Primary: Core (Rectus Abdominis, Obliques)
Secondary: Hip Flexors (Iliopsoas), Quadriceps (Rectus Femoris)

Equipment:
None

69. High Plank

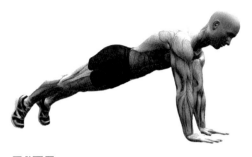 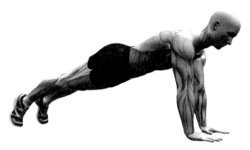

Instructions:

1. Begin on the floor on your hands and knees. Position your hands directly under your shoulders and your knees under your hips.

2. Extend your legs straight back, one at a time, coming onto the balls of your feet to form a straight line from your head to your heels. Your body should be in a high plank position.

3. Engage your core, glutes, and legs to maintain a straight body line. Keep your shoulders directly over your wrists.

4. Hold the plank position for the desired time, maintaining proper form and steady breathing.

Tips:

1. Keep your core engaged throughout the exercise to maintain stability and prevent sagging or arching of your back.

2. Ensure your hands are positioned directly under your shoulders to support your weight evenly.

3. Breathe steadily, inhaling through your nose and exhaling through your mouth to help maintain focus and endurance.

Active Muscles:
Primary: Core (Rectus Abdominis, Obliques)

Secondary: Shoulders (Deltoids)
Equipment:
None

70. Hollow Hold

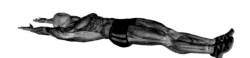

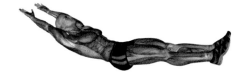

Instructions:

1. Lie on your back with your legs extended and your arms stretched overhead.

2. Engage your core and lift your shoulders and legs off the floor, keeping your lower back pressed into the floor. Your body should form a slight curve with your arms and legs elevated.

3. Hold this position, maintaining tension in your core and keeping your lower back flat against the floor.

4. Hold the position for the desired duration, then slowly lower your shoulders and legs back to the starting position.

Tips:

1. Ensure your shoulders and legs are lifted at the same height to create a balanced position.

2. Focus on steady breathing, inhaling through your nose and exhaling through your mouth to help maintain focus and endurance.

3. If the full hollow hold is too challenging, you can modify the position by bending your knees or keeping your arms by your sides.

Active Muscles:
Primary: Core (Rectus Abdominis, Obliques)

Secondary: Hip Flexors (Iliopsoas), Quadriceps (Rectus Femoris)
Equipment:
None

71. Leg Lift Circles

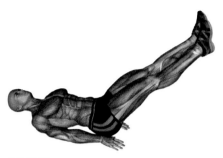

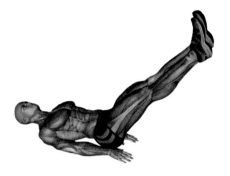

Instructions:

1. Lie on your back with your legs extended and your arms at your sides, palms facing down.

2. Lift both legs off the floor, about a foot above the floor, keeping your legs straight and your core engaged.

3. Begin to draw small circles in the air with both legs moving together in a controlled and steady motion. Perform the circles in one direction for a set number of repetitions.

4. Switch directions and draw circles with both legs in the opposite direction for the same number of repetitions. Lower your legs back to the starting position.

Tips:

1. Keep your legs as straight as possible to maximize the stretch and engagement in your hip flexors and quadriceps.

2. Perform the exercise on a comfortable, non-slip surface to prevent discomfort or injury.

3. If you find it challenging to keep your legs straight, you can start with smaller circles and gradually increase the size as you build strength and flexibility.

Active Muscles:
Primary: Core (Rectus Abdominis, Obliques), Hip Flexors (Iliopsoas)

Secondary: Quadriceps (Rectus Femoris)
Equipment:
None

72. Long Arm Crunches

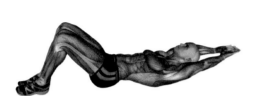 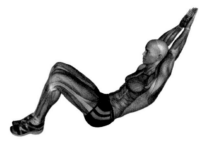

Instructions:

1. Lie flat on your back with your knees bent and your feet flat on the floor, hip-width apart. Extend your arms straight in line with your head, keeping them close to your ears and hands crossed over each other.

2. Engage your core and lift your upper body off the floor, with your arms following your torso line, until it forms a 45-degree angle with the floor.

3. Hold the top position for a second, squeezing your abdominal muscles.

4. Slowly lower your body back to the starting position with control. Repeat for the desired number of repetitions.

Tips:

1. Keep your arms straight and aligned with your ears to ensure proper form and avoid straining your neck.

2. Press your lower back firmly into the floor throughout the exercise to prevent lower back strain.

3. Use a comfortable, non-slip exercise mat to provide cushioning and prevent slipping during the movement.

Active Muscles:
Primary: Abdominals (Rectus Abdominis)

Secondary: Obliques (External Obliques, Internal Obliques)
Equipment:
None

73. Lying Leg Lift

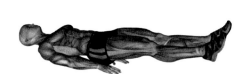 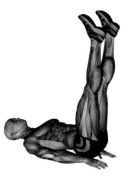

Instructions:

1. Lie flat on your back with your legs extended and raised a few inches off the floor, your arms at your sides, and your palms facing down firmly on the floor.

2. Engage your core muscles and press your lower back into the floor.

3. Keeping your legs straight, lift them up towards the ceiling until they are perpendicular to the floor.

4. Slowly lower your legs back to the starting position with control, stopping just before touching the floor. Repeat for the desired number of repetitions.

Tips:

1. Exhale as you lift your legs up and inhale as you lower them back down.

2. Keep your legs as straight as possible for maximum effectiveness.

3. Focus on engaging your abdominal muscles throughout the movement.

Active Muscles:
Primary: Abdominals (Rectus Abdominis)

Secondary: Hip Flexors (Iliopsoas)
Equipment:
None

74. Lying Leg Raise

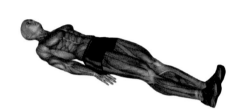 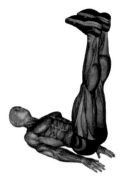

Instructions:

1. Lie flat on your back with your legs extended, your arms at your sides, and your palms facing down firmly on the floor.

2. Engage your core muscles and press your lower back into the floor.

3. Keeping your legs straight, lift them up towards the ceiling until they are perpendicular to the floor.

4. Slowly lower your legs back to the starting position with control, stopping when lightly touching the floor. Repeat for the desired number of repetitions.

Tips:

1. Exhale as you lift your legs up and inhale as you lower them back down.

2. Keep your legs as straight as possible for maximum effectiveness.

3. Focus on engaging your abdominal muscles throughout the movement.

Active Muscles:
Primary: Abdominals (Rectus Abdominis)

Secondary: Hip Flexors (Iliopsoas)
Equipment:
None

75. Mountain Climbers

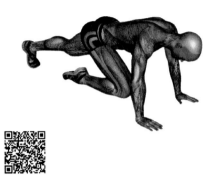
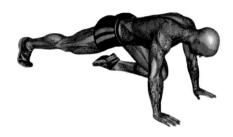

Instructions:
1. Begin in a plank position on your toes and hands, with your body in a straight line from head to heels.
2. Bend your right knee and bring it towards your right elbow, and stop when your knee is close to the elbow.
3. Return to the starting plank position, then repeat the movement on the opposite side.
4. Continue alternating sides for the desired number of repetitions.

Tips:
1. Ensure your movements are smooth and controlled to maintain form and avoid injury.
2. Maintain a steady breathing pattern, exhaling as you bring your knee towards your elbow and inhaling as you return to the plank position.
3. Keep your shoulders stable and your core engaged throughout the exercise to enhance effectiveness.

Active Muscles:
Primary: Core (Rectus Abdominis, Obliques)
Secondary: Shoulders (Deltoids)

Equipment:
None

76. Oblique Crunch

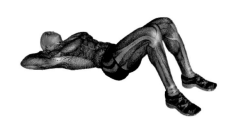

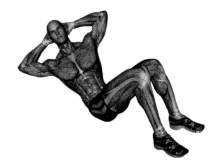

Instructions:

1. Lie on your back with your knees bent and feet flat on the floor. Place your hands behind your head, keeping your elbows wide.

2. Engage your core muscles and lift your upper back off the floor, rotating your abdomen to bring your right elbow towards the ceiling.

3. At the top of the movement, squeeze your obliques and slowly lower your upper back to the starting position with control.

4. Repeat for the desired repetitions, then switch sides to work the opposite obliques.

Tips:

1. Exhale as you lift and rotate your upper body, and inhale as you lower it back down.

2. Avoid pulling on your neck with your hands; let your abs do the work.

3. Focus on engaging your oblique muscles throughout the movement.

Active Muscles:
Primary: Obliques (External Obliques, Internal Obliques)

Secondary: Abdominals (Rectus Abdominis), Hip Flexors (Iliopsoas)
Equipment:
None

77. Plank Cross Knee Drive

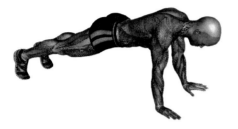
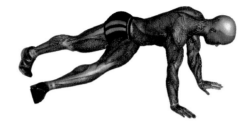

Instructions:

1. Begin in a plank position with your hands directly under your shoulders and your body forming a straight line from head to heels.

2. Lift your right knee and drive it towards your left elbow, and straighten your leg as much as possible, twisting your torso slightly to the left as you do so.

3. Return your right leg to the starting plank position.

4. Repeat the movement with your left knee, driving it towards your right elbow. Alternate sides for the desired number of repetitions.

Tips:

1. Keep your core engaged throughout the exercise to maintain stability and support your lower back.

2. Move slowly and with control to maximize muscle engagement and prevent injury.

3. Focus on steady breathing, exhaling as you drive your knee towards your elbow and inhaling as you return to the starting position.

Active Muscles:
Primary: Core (Rectus Abdominis, Obliques)

Secondary: Shoulders (Deltoids), Hip Flexors (Iliopsoas)
Equipment:
None

78. Plank Jack

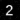

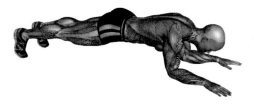
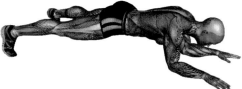

Instructions:

1. Begin in a plank position with your elbows directly under your shoulders and your body forming a straight line from head to heels.

2. Jump your feet out to the sides, slightly wider than shoulder-width apart, while keeping your upper body stable.

3. Quickly jump your feet back together to return to the starting plank position.

4. Continue jumping your feet in and out for the desired repetitions or duration.

Tips:

1. Move quickly but with control to maximize muscle engagement and prevent injury.

2. Maintain a neutral head position, looking slightly ahead of your hands, to keep your neck aligned with your spine.

3. Ensure your body stays straight, avoiding sagging hips or raised buttocks.

Active Muscles:
Primary: Core (Rectus Abdominis, Obliques)
Secondary: Shoulders (Deltoids), Hip Flexors (Iliopsoas), Quadriceps (Rectus Femoris)

Equipment:
None

79. Plank Knee Tucks

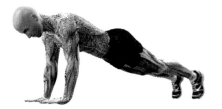
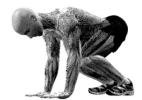

Instructions:

1. Begin in a plank position with your hands directly under your shoulders and your body forming a straight line from head to heels.

2. Quickly jump both knees towards your chest, landing with both feet flat on the floor underneath you.

3. Immediately jump your feet back to the starting plank position.

4. Continue jumping your feet in and out for the desired number of repetitions.

Tips:

1. Use controlled, explosive movements to quickly bring your knees to your chest and return to the plank position.

2. Ensure your shoulders remain directly over your wrists to maintain alignment and reduce strain on your shoulders.

3. Keep your hips level throughout the movement to maintain proper form and avoid sagging or raising your hips.

Active Muscles:
Primary: Core (Rectus Abdominis, Obliques)

Secondary: Shoulders (Deltoids), Hip Flexors (Iliopsoas), Quadriceps (Rectus Femoris)
Equipment:
None

The Ultimate Exercise Guide: Abdominals Edition - 1st Edition

80. Plank On Elbows

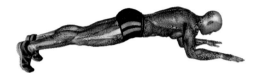

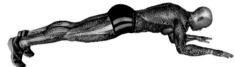

Instructions:

1. Begin by lying face down on the floor. Place your elbows directly under your shoulders and your forearms flat on the floor, parallel to each other.

2. Engage your core and lift your body off the floor, forming a straight line from your head to your heels. Your elbows and toes should support your body weight.

3. Hold this position, keeping your core tight and your body straight. Avoid letting your hips sag or rise too high.

4. Maintain the plank position for the desired time, focusing on your form and breathing steadily.

Tips:

1. Engage your core throughout the exercise to maintain stability and support your lower back.

2. Keep your body in a straight line from head to heels, avoiding any sagging or lifting of the hips.

3. Keep your shoulders directly above your elbows to maintain proper alignment and reduce strain on your shoulders.

Active Muscles:
Primary: Core (Rectus Abdominis, Obliques)

Secondary: Shoulders (Deltoids), Lower Back (Erector Spinae)
Equipment:
None

81. Plank Reach Through

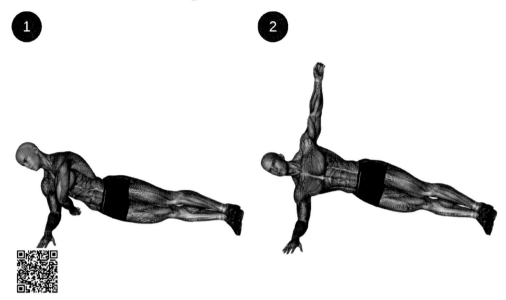

Instructions:

1. Begin in a side plank position on your right side with your right elbow supporting your body, your left arm raised vertically towards the ceiling, and your body forming a straight line from head to heels.

2. Lower your left arm, reaching it under and across your torso while slightly lowering your hips.

3. Return your left arm to the starting position, lifting your hips back to the straight line.

4. Repeat for the desired number of repetitions, then switch to the left side and repeat the movement with your right arm.

Tips:

1. Engage your core throughout the exercise to maintain stability and support your lower back.

2. Ensure your supporting arm or elbow is directly under your shoulder to maintain proper alignment and reduce strain.

3. Keep your hips stable and aligned with your body, avoiding excessive rotation.

Active Muscles:
Primary: Obliques (External Obliques, Internal Obliques), Abdominals (Rectus Abdominis)

Secondary: Shoulders (Deltoids), Upper Back (Trapezius)
Equipment:
None

82. Raised Leg Crunch

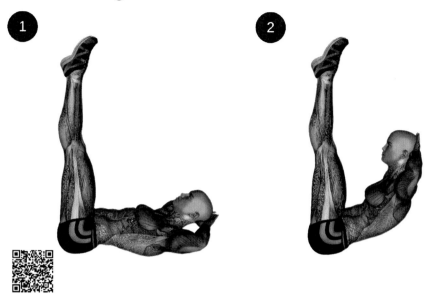

Instructions:

1. Lie on your back with your legs straight and vertical to the floor. Place your hands behind your head, with your elbows pointing outwards.

2. Engage your core and lift your shoulders off the floor, bringing your chest towards your knees.

3. Hold the top position for a second, squeezing your abdominal muscles.

4. Lower your shoulders back to the starting position with control. Repeat for the desired number of repetitions

Tips:

1. Avoid pulling on your neck with your hands; use your abdominal muscles to lift your shoulders.

2. Breathe steadily, exhaling as you lift your shoulders and inhaling as you lower them.

3. Keep your lower back pressed against the floor to prevent strain and maintain proper form.

Active Muscles:
Primary: Abdominals (Rectus Abdominis)

Secondary: Hip Flexors (Iliopsoas)
Equipment:
None

83. Reverse Crunch With Kick Out

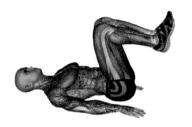
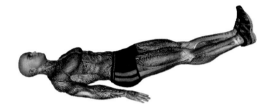

Instructions:

1. Lie on your back with your knees bent and feet flat on the floor. Place your arms by your sides, palms facing down for stability.

2. Lift your legs off the floor, bending your knees at a 90-degree angle so that your thighs are perpendicular to the floor and your lower legs are parallel to the floor.

3. Extend your legs straight out, keeping them off the floor to perform a kick-out.

4. Bend your knees back to the starting position and engage your core to lift your hips off the floor, curling your knees towards your chest. Lower your hips back to the starting position. Repeat for the desired number of repetitions.

Tips:

1. Avoid using momentum to lift your hips; focus on using your abdominal muscles.

2. Perform the exercise on a comfortable, non-slip surface to ensure safety and reduce discomfort.

3. Keep your head and shoulders relaxed on the floor to avoid straining your neck.

Active Muscles:
Primary: Abdominals (Rectus Abdominis)

Secondary: Hip Flexors (Iliopsoas), Obliques (External Obliques, Internal Obliques)
Equipment:
None

84. Reverse Crunch

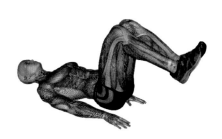

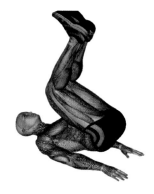

Instructions:

1. Lie on your back with your knees bent and feet flat on the floor. Place your arms by your sides, palms facing down for stability.

2. Lift your legs off the floor, bending your knees at a 90-degree angle so that your thighs are perpendicular to the floor and your lower legs are parallel to the floor.

3. Engage your core and lift your hips off the floor, curling your knees towards your chest.

4. Slowly lower your hips back to the starting position, keeping your knees bent at a 90-degree angle. Repeat for the desired number of repetitions.

Tips:

1. Avoid using momentum to lift your hips; focus on using your abdominal muscles.

2. Breathe steadily, exhaling as you lift your hips and inhaling as you lower them back down.

3. Keep your head and shoulders relaxed on the floor to avoid straining your neck.

Active Muscles:
Primary: Abdominals (Rectus Abdominis)

Secondary: Hip Flexors (Iliopsoas), Obliques (External Obliques, Internal Obliques)
Equipment:
None

85. Russian Twist

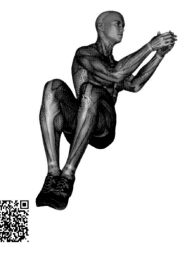

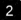

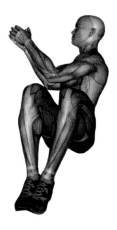

Instructions:
1. Sit on the floor with your knees bent and feet flat on the floor. Lean back slightly so that your torso forms a V-shape with your thighs.
2. Clasp your hands together in front of your chest.
3. Rotate your torso to the right, bringing your hands opposite your right hip.
4. Rotate back through the center and to the left, bringing your hands opposite your left hip. Continue alternating sides for the desired number of repetitions.

Tips:
1. Move your torso, not your arms, to ensure you engage your oblique muscles.
2. Breathe steadily, exhaling as you rotate to each side and inhaling as you return to the center.
3. Keep your back straight and avoid hunching your shoulders to maintain proper form.

Active Muscles:
Primary: Obliques (External Obliques, Internal Obliques)
Secondary: Abdominals (Rectus Abdominis), Hip Flexors (Iliopsoas)

Equipment:
None

86. Scissors Kick

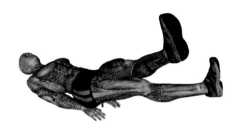

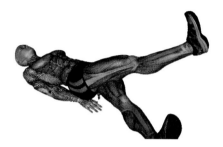

Instructions:

1. Lie on your back with your legs extended and your arms by your sides, palms facing down.

2. Lift both legs off the floor a few inches, keeping them straight.

3. Alternately cross your legs over each other in a scissor-like motion. Move your right leg over your left leg and then switch, bringing your left leg over your right leg.

4. Continue alternating legs in a controlled manner for the desired number of repetitions or duration.

Tips:

1. Ensure your lower back remains pressed against the floor to avoid strain and maintain proper form.

2. Move your legs slowly and with control to maximize muscle engagement and prevent injury.

3. Perform the exercise on a comfortable, non-slip surface to ensure safety and reduce discomfort.

Active Muscles:
Primary: Abdominals (Rectus Abdominis)

Secondary: Hip Flexors (Iliopsoas), Inner Thigh (Adductors), Outer Thigh (Abductors)
Equipment:
None

87. Seated Floor Crunches

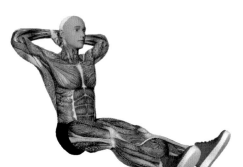

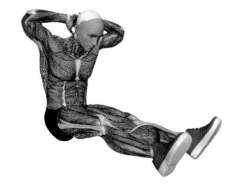

Instructions:
1. Sit on the floor with your legs extended straight out in front of you, forming an L-shape with your torso.
2. Place your hands behind your head without pulling on your neck, elbows facing outwards.
3. Engage your core and bend your torso towards your thighs, performing a crunch while keeping your legs straight.
4. Bring your torso back to the starting position with control. Repeat for the desired number of repetitions.

Tips:
1. Avoid pulling on your neck with your hands; use your abdominal muscles to lower your torso.
2. Breathe steadily, exhaling as you lift your torso and inhaling as you lower it back down.
3. Keep your legs straight and flat on the floor to maintain stability during the exercise.

Active Muscles:
Primary: Abdominals (Rectus Abdominis)
Secondary: Hip Flexors (Iliopsoas)

Equipment:
None

88. Seated Flutter Kicks

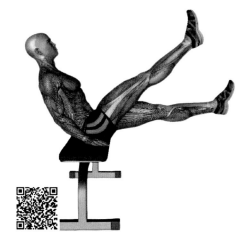 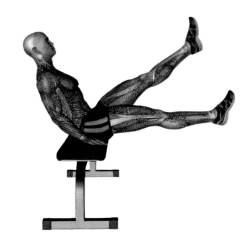

Instructions:

1. Sit on a bench with your legs extended straight out. Lean back slightly, supporting yourself by gripping the sides of the bench.

2. Lift both legs off the bench, keeping them straight.

3. Begin the flutter kicks by alternately raising and lower-ing your legs in a scissor-like motion, moving your right leg up while your left leg moves down and vice versa.

4. Continue the flutter kicks for the desired repetitions or duration, keeping your core engaged and your movements controlled.

Tips:

1. Keep your back straight and avoid rounding your shoulders to maintain proper form.

2. Perform the exercise on a stable, non-slip bench to ensure safety and prevent slipping.

3. If you are new to this exercise, start with a smaller range of motion and gradually increase it as you build strength.

Active Muscles:
Primary: Abdominals (Rectus Abdominis)

Secondary: Hip Flexors (Iliopsoas), Obliques (External Obliques, Internal Obliques)
Equipment:
None

89. Seated V Up

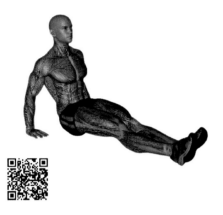

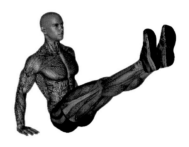

Instructions:
1. Sit on the floor with your legs extended straight in front of you and your arms placed on the floor slightly behind you for support.
2. Engage your core and lift your torso off the floor, bringing your knees towards your chest to form a V shape with your body.
3. Hold the top position for a second, squeezing your abdominal muscles.
4. Lower your legs and torso back to the starting position with control. Repeat for the desired number of repetitions.

Tips:
1. Breathe steadily, exhaling as you lift into the V position and inhaling as you lower back down.
2. Avoid using momentum to lift your legs and torso; focus on using your abdominal muscles.
3. Keep your back straight and avoid rounding your shoulders to maintain proper form.

Active Muscles:
Primary: Abdominals (Rectus Abdominis)

Secondary: Hip Flexors (Iliopsoas)
Equipment:
None

90. Side Plank Oblique Crunch

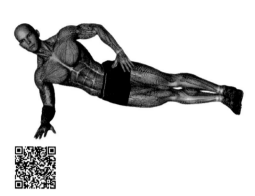

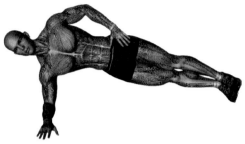

Instructions:

1. Begin in a side plank position on your right side, with your legs extended straight and stacked on each other. Prop yourself up on your right elbow, keeping your elbow directly under your shoulder. Place your left hand on your hip.

2. Engage your core and lift your hips off the floor, forming a straight line from your head to your feet.

3. Lower your hips towards the floor without touching it, then raise them back up to the starting position, squeezing your obliques at the top.

4. Repeat for the desired number of repetitions, then switch to the other side and perform the exercise on your left side.

Tips:

1. Keep your core engaged throughout the exercise to maintain balance and stability.

2. Move your hips slowly and with control to maximize muscle engagement and prevent injury.

3. Breathe steadily, exhaling as you lift your hips and inhaling as you lower them.

Active Muscles:
Primary: Obliques (External Obliques, Internal Obliques)

Secondary: Abdominals (Rectus Abdominis), Shoulders (Deltoids)
Equipment:
None

91. Side Plank With Hip Lift

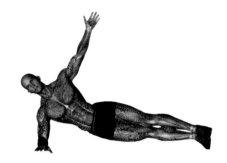 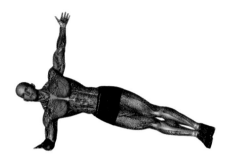

Instructions:

1. Begin in a side plank position on your right side, with your legs extended straight and stacked on each other. Prop yourself up on your right elbow, keeping your elbow directly under your shoulder. Raise your left arm straight toward the ceiling.
2. Engage your core and lift your hips off the floor, forming a straight line from your head to your feet.
3. Once in the top position, perform two small controlled bounces with your hips, lifting them slightly higher each time.
4. Lower your hips back to the floor without touching it and repeat the steps for the desired number of repetitions, then switch to the other side and perform the exercise on your left side.

Tips:

1. Move your hips slowly and with control to maximize muscle engagement and prevent injury.
2. Breathe steadily, exhaling as you lift your hips and inhaling as you lower them.
3. Ensure your elbow is directly under your shoulder to support your upper body.

Active Muscles:
Primary: Obliques (External Obliques, Internal Obliques)

Secondary: Abdominals (Rectus Abdominis), Shoulders (Deltoids)
Equipment:
None

92. Side Plank

 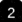

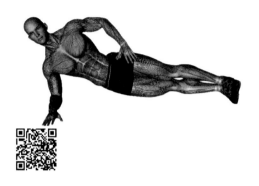 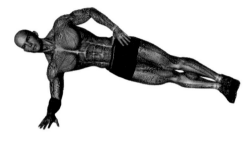

Instructions:

1. Lie on your right side with your legs extended straight and stacked on each other. Prop yourself up on your right elbow, keeping your elbow directly under your shoulder.

2. Engage your core and lift your hips off the floor, forming a straight line from your head to your feet.

3. Hold the position for the desired duration, keeping your body straight and your core tight.

4. Slowly lower your hips back to the starting position with control. Repeat on the other side and follow the same steps.

Tips:

1. Ensure your elbow is directly under your shoulder to support your upper body.

2. Focus on keeping your head in line with your spine to prevent neck strain.

3. Maintain a straight body line, avoiding any sagging or lifting of the hips.

Active Muscles:
Primary: Obliques (External Obliques, Internal Obliques)

Secondary: Abdominals (Rectus Abdominis), Shoulders (Deltoids)
Equipment:
None

93. Side To Side Punch

1

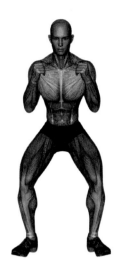

2

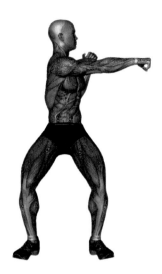

Instructions:

1. Stand upright with your feet wider than shoulder-width apart and your knees slightly bent. Hold your fists up in front of your face in a guard position.

2. Rotate your torso to the left as you punch across your body with your right hand, extending your arm fully. Keep your legs and hips stationary.

3. Quickly return to the starting position, then rotate your torso to the right as you punch across your body with your left hand.

4. Continue alternating punches from side to side for the desired duration or number of repetitions, maintaining a steady rhythm and controlled movements.

Tips:

1. Focus on rotating your torso to generate power in your punches while keeping your legs and hips stationary.

2. Breathe steadily, exhaling as you punch and inhaling as you return to the starting position.

3. Keep your fists up in a guard position when not punching to simulate a defensive stance.

Active Muscles:
Primary: Core (Rectus Abdominis, Obliques)

Secondary: Shoulders (Deltoids), Arms (Biceps, Triceps)
Equipment:
None

94. Sit-Ups

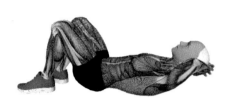

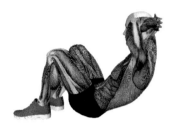

Instructions:

1. Lie on your back with your knees bent and feet flat on the floor, hip-width apart. Place your hands behind your head.

2. Engage your core and lift your upper body off the floor, curling your chest towards your knees.

3. Continue lifting your torso until you are in a sitting position with your chest close to your knees.

4. Slowly lower your upper body back to the starting position with control. Repeat for the desired number of repetitions.

Tips:

1. Keep your core engaged throughout the exercise to maximize muscle engagement and support your lower back.

2. Move your body slowly and with control to avoid using momentum and to prevent injury.

3. Breathe steadily, exhaling as you lift your torso and inhaling as you lower it back down.

Active Muscles:
Primary: Abdominals (Rectus Abdominis)

Secondary: Hip Flexors (Iliopsoas)
Equipment:
None

95. Spider Plank

1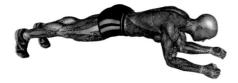

2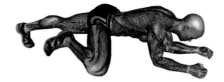

Instructions:

1. Begin in a standard plank position with your forearms on the floor, elbows directly under your shoulders, and your body forming a straight line from head to heels. Engage your core and keep your feet hip-width apart.

2. Lift your right foot off the floor and bring your right knee towards your right elbow, keeping your hips level and your core tight.

3. Return your right foot to the starting position, maintaining a stable plank position.

4. Repeat the movement with your left leg, bringing your left knee towards your left elbow. Continue alternating legs for the desired duration or number of repetitions.

Tips:

1. Breathe steadily throughout the exercise, exhaling as you bring your knee towards your elbow and inhaling as you return to the starting position.

2. Focus on keeping your hips level and avoiding excessive torso rotation.

3. Use a mat to cushion your forearms and feet for added comfort.

Active Muscles:
Primary: Core (Rectus Abdominis, Obliques)

Secondary: Shoulders (Deltoids), Hip Flexors (Iliopsoas)
Equipment:
None

96. Standing Oblique Crunch

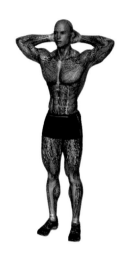

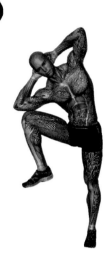

Instructions:
1. Stand with your feet shoulder-width apart, placing your hands behind your head with your elbows out to the sides. Engage your core and maintain an upright posture.
2. Lift your right knee towards your right elbow while bending your torso to the right to bring your elbow and knee closer together.
3. Return to the starting position by lowering your right leg and straightening your torso.
4. Repeat the movement on the left side, lifting your left knee towards your left elbow. Continue alternating sides for the desired number of repetitions.

Tips:
1. Breathe steadily: exhale as you crunch to the side, and inhale as you return to the starting position.
2. Ensure your standing leg remains slightly bent to maintain balance.
3. Keep your back straight and avoid leaning forward or backward during the exercise.

Active Muscles:
Primary: Abdominals (Obliques)
Secondary: Abdominals (Rectus Abdominis, Transverse Abdominis), Hip Flexors (Iliopsoas), Shoulders (Deltoids), Quadriceps (Quadriceps Femoris)
Equipment:
None

97. Star Crunches

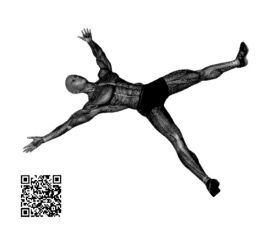 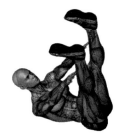

Instructions:

1. Lie flat on your back with your arms and legs extended diagonally to form an "X" shape. Keep your core engaged and your lower back pressed into the floor.

2. Crunch your abdominal muscles to lift your shoulders and legs off the floor and lift your arms and legs towards each other, reaching your hands towards your ankles.

3. Lower your arms and legs back to the starting position with control.

4. Repeat the movement for the desired number of repetitions.

Tips:

1. Breathe steadily: exhale as you lift your arm and leg, and inhale as you return to the starting position.

2. Focus on using your abdominal muscles to lift your arms and legs off the floor.

3. Use a mat to provide cushioning and support for your back.

Active Muscles:
Primary: Abdominals (Rectus Abdominis, Obliques)
Secondary: Hip Flexors (Iliopsoas), Quadriceps (Quadriceps Femoris)

Equipment:
None

98. V Up

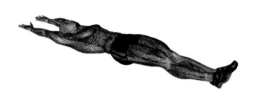

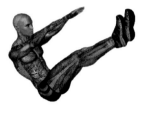

Instructions:

1. Lie flat on your back on the floor with your legs and arms extended so that your body forms a straight line.

2. Simultaneously lift your legs and torso off the floor, reaching your hands towards your feet to form a 'V' shape with your body.

3. Squeeze your abdominal muscles at the top of the movement, ensuring your hands reach towards your feet.

4. Slowly lower your legs and torso back to the starting position with control. Repeat for the desired number of repetitions.

Tips:

1. Breathe steadily: exhale as you lift into the 'V' position and inhale as you lower back down.

2. Avoid using momentum to lift your legs and torso; focus on using your abdominal muscles.

3. Keep your legs and arms straight throughout the movement for maximum effectiveness.

Active Muscles:
Primary: Abdominals (Rectus Abdominis, Obliques)

Secondary: Hip Flexors (Iliopsoas), Quadriceps (Quadriceps Femoris)
Equipment:
None

99. Wind Wipers

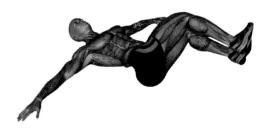

Instructions:

1. Lie on your back with your arms extended out to the sides for stability. Lift your legs up towards the ceiling and keep them bent at 90 degrees.

2. Lower your knees to the right side, keeping them bent and together until they are just above the floor.

3. Raise your knees back to the center position, then lower them to the left side until they are just above the floor.

4. Repeat the movement, alternating sides, for the desired number of repetitions.

Tips:

1. Use a mat or soft surface to support your back and prevent discomfort.

2. Avoid using momentum to move your legs; focus on using your abdominal and oblique muscles.

3. Keep your shoulders flat on the floor to maintain stability and proper form.

Active Muscles:
Primary: Obliques (External Obliques), Abdominals (Rectus Abdominis)

Secondary: Hip Flexors (Iliopsoas), Lower Back (Erector Spinae)
Equipment:
None

CHAPTER 3

FREE WEIGHTS

What Are Free Weight Exercises?

Free weight exercises involve using external weights, such as dumbbells, barbells, specialized bars like EZ bars, kettlebells, or weight plates to create resistance during workouts. Unlike machines, which guide your movement, free weights allow for a full range of motion and require stabilizing muscles to control the weight. Examples of free-weight movements include deadlifts, bench presses, and dumbbell curls. Free weights can be used for various training goals, from building muscle and strength to improving balance and coordination, making them a versatile tool in any fitness routine.

Why Use Free Weight Exercises?

Free weight exercises offer unique benefits by challenging large muscle groups and smaller stabilizing muscles that help balance and control. This makes them especially effective for building functional strength and improving overall muscle development. Because free weights allow for greater flexibility in movement, they also enable you to target specific muscles and easily adjust the difficulty of your workout. Whether aiming for increased strength, muscle hypertrophy, or enhanced athletic performance, free weights provide the versatility and challenge needed to progress at any fitness level.

What Are Barbell Exercises?

Barbell exercises involve using a long bar loaded with weight plates to add resistance during workouts. Unlike dumbbells, which allow for independent arm movement, barbells are held with both hands, providing a more stable base for lifting heavier weights. Barbell exercises often focus on compound movements, such as squats, deadlifts, and bench presses, which engage multiple muscle groups simultaneously. This makes barbells ideal for building overall strength, power, and muscle mass, whether training for performance, muscle growth, or general fitness.

Why Use Barbell Exercises?

Barbell exercises offer distinct advantages by allowing you to lift heavier weights and perform fundamental compound movements that build full-body strength. Because barbells engage multiple muscle groups at once, they are incredibly efficient for increasing muscle mass and improving overall functional strength. The ability to progressively add weight makes barbells especially effective for tracking and achieving strength goals. Whether focusing on powerlifting, bodybuilding, or improving your athletic performance, barbells provide the resistance and stability needed to take your strength training to the next level.

100. Barbell Rollout

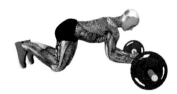 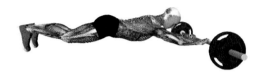

Instructions:

1. Begin by kneeling on the floor with a barbell in front of you. Grab the barbell with an overhand grip (palms facing down), hands shoulder-width apart.

2. Slowly roll the barbell forward, extending your arms and allowing your body to move forward.

3. Roll out as far as possible while maintaining control and a neutral spine. Your arms should be fully extended, and your body should be in a straight line from your head to your knees.

4. Engage your core and pull the barbell back to the starting position. Repeat for the desired number of repetitions.

Tips:

1. Maintain a strong core throughout the movement to stabilize your spine and prevent injury.

2. Keep your back flat and avoid letting your hips sag to ensure proper form.

3. Control the rolling motion to maximize muscle engagement and prevent strain.

Active Muscles:
Primary: Abdominals (Rectus Abdominis), Obliques (External Obliques)

Secondary: Shoulders (Deltoids), Upper Back (Trapezius)
Equipment:
Barbell

101. Barbell Seated Twist On Exercise Ball

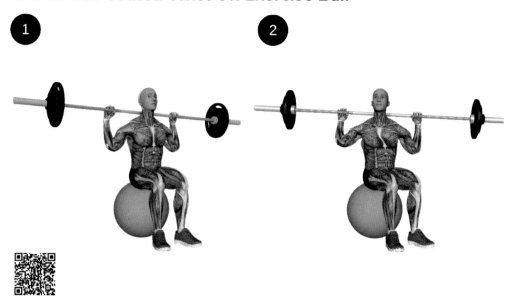

Instructions:

1. Sit on an exercise ball with your feet flat on the floor, holding a barbell across your upper back with an overhand grip, hands slightly wider than shoulder-width apart. Keep your back straight and your core engaged.

2. Begin by rotating your torso to the right, keeping your hips and lower body stationary. Rotate until you feel a stretch in your obliques.

3. Reverse the movement, rotating your torso to the left, keeping your hips and lower body stationary.

4. Repeat the rotation to both sides for the desired number of repetitions.

Tips:

1. Engage your core muscles to stabilize your spine and maintain proper form.

2. Maintain an upright posture to avoid straining your lower back.

3. Use a weight that allows proper form and control throughout the exercise to prevent strain or injury.

Active Muscles:
Primary: Obliques (External Obliques, Internal Obliques)

Secondary: Abdominals (Rectus Abdominis), Lower Back (Erector Spinae)
Equipment:
Exercise Ball, Barbell

102. Barbell Seated Twist

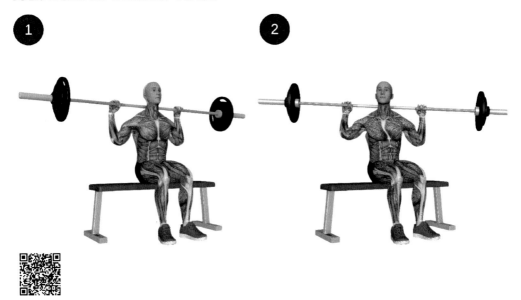

Instructions:

1. Sit on a bench with your feet flat on the floor, holding a barbell across your upper back with an overhand grip, hands slightly wider than shoulder-width apart. Keep your back straight and your core engaged.

2. Begin by rotating your torso to the right, keeping your hips and lower body stationary. Rotate until you feel a stretch in your obliques.

3. Reverse the movement, rotating your torso to the left, keeping your hips and lower body stationary.

4. Repeat the rotation to both sides for the desired number of repetitions.

Tips:

1. Engage your core muscles to stabilize your spine and maintain proper form.

2. Maintain an upright posture to avoid straining your lower back.

3. Use a weight that allows proper form and control throughout the exercise to prevent strain or injury.

Active Muscles:
Primary: Obliques (External Obliques, Internal Obliques)

Secondary: Abdominals (Rectus Abdominis), Lower Back (Erector Spinae)
Equipment:
Bench, Barbell

103. Barbell Side Bends

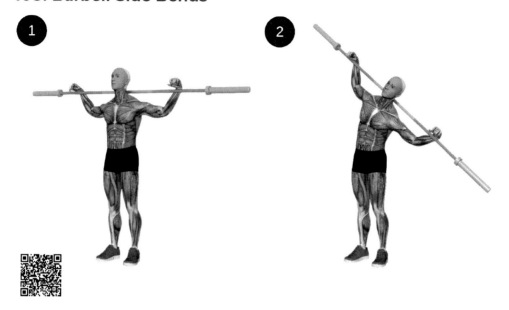

Instructions:

1. Stand with your feet shoulder-width apart, holding a barbell across your upper back with an overhand grip, hands slightly wider than shoulder-width apart. Keep your back straight and your core engaged.

2. Lean to the right side by bending at the waist, lowering your torso as far as possible.

3. Return to the starting position by engaging your oblique muscles and straightening your torso.

4. Repeat the movement to the left side. Continue alternating sides for the desired number of repetitions.

Tips:

1. Avoid twisting your torso to focus on the side bend during the movement.

2. Breathe steadily, exhaling as you bend to each side and inhaling as you return to the center.

3. Keep your movements slow and controlled to maximize muscle engagement and prevent injury.

Active Muscles:
Primary: Obliques (External Obliques, Internal Obliques)

Secondary: Abdominals (Rectus Abdominis), Lower Back (Erector Spinae)
Equipment:
Barbell

104. Barbell Standing Twist

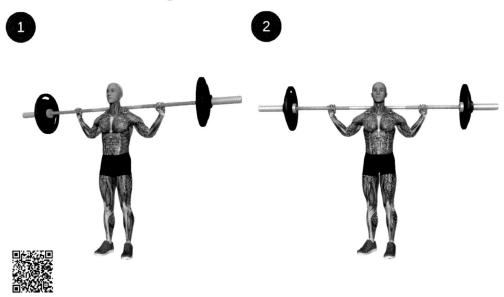

Instructions:
1. Stand with your feet shoulder-width apart, holding a barbell across your upper back with an overhand grip, hands slightly wider than shoulder-width apart.

2. Rotate your torso to the right, keeping your hips and knees aligned with the movement.

3. Rotate back to the center position with control, then twist your torso to the left.

4. Continue alternating sides, repeating for the desired number of repetitions.

Tips:
1. Rotate your torso, not just your arms, to engage your oblique muscles effectively.

2. Breathe steadily, exhaling as you twist and inhaling as you return to the center position.

3. Use a weight that allows proper form and control throughout the exercise to prevent strain or injury.

Active Muscles:
Primary: Obliques (External Obliques, Internal Obliques)

Secondary: Abdominals (Rectus Abdominis), Lower Back (Erector Spinae)

Equipment:
Barbell

What Are Dumbbell Exercises?

Dumbbell exercises involve using a pair of handheld free weights to add resistance during workouts. Unlike machines, which control the path of your movement, dumbbells allow for a natural, unrestricted range of motion and engage stabilizing muscles to maintain balance and control. Dumbbells can be used in a variety of movements, from basic curls and presses to compound lifts like squats and lunges. Whether your goal is muscle growth, strength enhancement, or boosting endurance, dumbbells are a highly versatile piece of equipment for any fitness routine.

Why Use Dumbbell Exercises?

Dumbbell exercises provide unique advantages by targeting both major muscle groups and smaller stabilizers that help improve coordination and balance. The versatility of dumbbells allows you to perform a wide range of exercises that can be easily adapted to fit your fitness level. Whether you're looking to build strength, increase muscle size, or improve functional movement, dumbbells give you the freedom to isolate muscles or engage multiple muscle groups in a single exercise. Their adaptability also allows you to scale workouts by adjusting the weight or exercise complexity, making dumbbells an essential tool for achieving continuous progress at any stage of your fitness journey.

105. Decline Bench Oblique Crunches Dumbbells

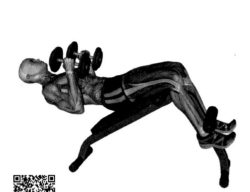
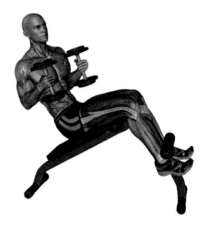

Instructions:

1. Secure your feet at the end of a decline bench and lie back with your knees bent. Hold a dumbbell in each hand close to your chest.

2. Engage your core and lift your upper body off the bench by contracting your abdominal muscles while twisting your torso to the right.

3. Squeeze your obliques at the top of the movement, ensuring the contraction is felt along the side of your abdomen.

4. Slowly lower your upper body back to the starting position and repeat the movement, twisting your torso to the left. Continue alternating sides for the desired number of repetitions.

Tips:

1. Breathe out as you twist and crunch, and breathe in as you return to the starting position.

2. Ensure your lower back stays in contact with the bench to support your spine.

3. Use a weight that challenges you but allows you to maintain proper form.

4. Keep your feet securely anchored to the bench to stabilize your body throughout the exercise.

Active Muscles:
Primary: Obliques (Internal and External Obliques), Abdominals (Rectus Abdominis)

Secondary: Biceps (Biceps Brachii), Hip Flexors (Iliopsoas)
Equipment:
Decline Bench, Dumbbells

106. Decline Sit Ups Dumbbells

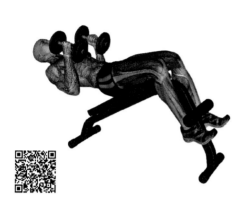
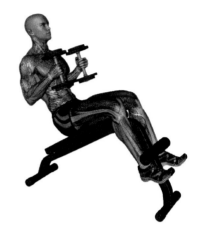

Instructions:

1. Secure your feet at the end of a decline bench and lie back with your knees bent. Hold a dumbbell in each hand close to your chest.

2. Engage your core and lift your upper body off the bench by contracting your abdominal muscles.

3. Continue lifting your upper body until you are seated, ensuring that the contraction is felt in your abs.

4. Slowly lower your upper body back to the starting position with control. Repeat for the desired number of repetitions.

Tips:

1. Focus on using your abdominal muscles to lift your body rather than relying on momentum.

2. Breathe out as you sit up and breathe in as you return to the starting position.

3. Keep your feet securely anchored to the bench to stabilize your body throughout the exercise.

Active Muscles:
Primary: Abdominals (Rectus Abdominis)

Secondary: Biceps (Biceps Brachii), Hip Flexors (Iliopsoas)
Equipment:
Decline Bench, Dumbbells

107. Dumbbell Crunch Hold With Legs Off

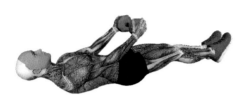 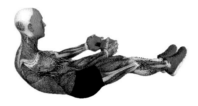

Instructions:

1. Lie flat on your back with your knees straight, and your legs lifted off the floor almost parallel to the floor, holding a dumbbell with both hands extended just over your hips.

2. Engage your core and lift your shoulder blades off the floor, performing a crunch while pushing the dumbbell over your thighs.

3. Hold the crunch position for a few seconds, ensuring your abs are fully engaged, and your lower back remains pressed into the floor.

4. Slowly lower your shoulders back to the floor, maintaining control of the dumbbell throughout the movement. Repeat for the desired number of repetitions.

Tips:

1. Breathe out as you lift your shoulders off the floor and inhale as you lower them back down.

2. Focus on engaging your core muscles throughout the exercise for maximum effectiveness.

3. Start with a lighter weight to ensure proper form and gradually increase as you become more comfortable.

Active Muscles:
Primary: Abdominals (Rectus Abdominis)

Secondary: Biceps (Biceps Brachii), Hip Flexors (Iliopsoas)
Equipment:
Dumbbells

108. Dumbbell Decline Overhead Sit-Up

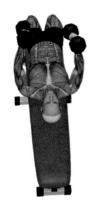

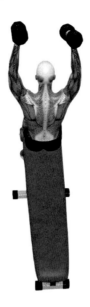

Instructions:

1. Begin by lying on a decline bench with your feet secured, holding a dumbbell in each hand extended overhead.

2. Slowly lift your shoulders and upper back off the bench while simultaneously raising the dumbbells above your head.

3. Continue to lift your torso until you are upright with the dumbbell directly above your head.

4. Slowly lower yourself back down to the starting position, keeping the dumbbells extended overhead.

Tips:

1. Keep your neck in a neutral position to avoid strain.

2. Focus on a smooth and controlled motion to maximize core engagement.

3. Avoid using momentum to lift yourself; rely on your core muscles.

Active Muscles:
Primary: Abdominals (Rectus Abdominis)
Secondary: Hip Flexors (Iliopsoas), Shoulders (Deltoids), Chest (Pectoralis Major)

Equipment:
Decline Bench, Dumbbells

109. Dumbbell Decline Sit-Up

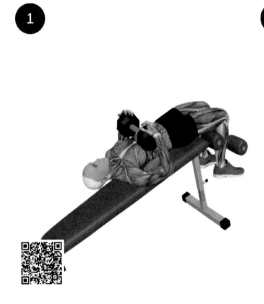

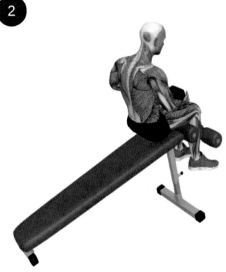

Instructions:

1. Lie on a decline bench with your feet securely positioned under the footpads. Hold a dumbbell with both hands against your chest.

2. Lift your upper body towards your knees, keeping the dumbbell close to your chest.

3. Sit up fully until your back is straight, then slowly lower your upper body back to the starting position.

4. Repeat the exercise for the desired number of repetitions.

Tips:

1. Keep the dumbbell close to your chest throughout the exercise to maintain balance.

2. Focus on engaging your abdominal muscles, not using momentum.

3. Keep your head and neck aligned with your spine to avoid strain.

Active Muscles:
Primary: Abdominals (Rectus Abdominis)
Secondary: Hip Flexors (Iliopsoas)

Equipment:
Decline Bench, Dumbbell

110. Dumbbell Diagonal Chop

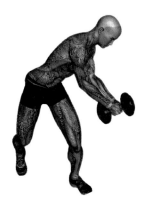

Instructions:

1. Stand with your feet shoulder-width apart, holding a dumbbell with both hands extended opposite your chest.

2. Rotate your torso and lower the dumbbell diagonally across your body to the left side, extending your arms fully as you reach downward while pivoting your feet towards your left side.

3. In a controlled motion, bring the dumbbell back up to the starting position, reversing the diagonal path.

4. Repeat the movement for the desired number of repetitions, then switch sides and repeat.

Tips:

1. Rotate your torso and pivot your feet to allow for a full range of motion.

2. Maintain a firm grip on the dumbbell to ensure control.

3. Perform the movement in a controlled manner to avoid swinging the dumbbell.

Active Muscles:
Primary: Obliques (External Oblique, Internal Oblique)
Secondary: Shoulders (Deltoids)

Equipment:
Dumbbell

111. Dumbbell Overhead Sit-Up

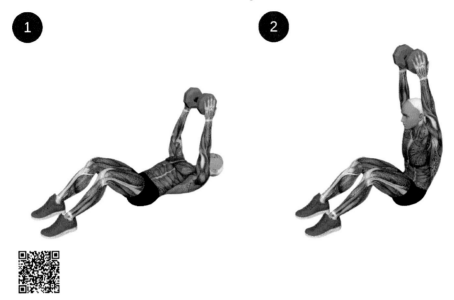

Instructions:
1. Lie on your back with your legs bent and feet flat on the floor. Hold a dumbbell in both hands, extending your arms straight overhead with your palms facing each other.
2. Engage your core and lift your upper body off the floor into a sitting position, keeping the dumbbell directly overhead.
3. Slowly lower your upper body back to the starting position, maintaining control and keeping the dumbbell overhead.
4. Repeat the movement for the desired number of repetitions.

Tips:
1. Ensure the dumbbell remains directly overhead and aligned with your shoulders during the entire movement.
2. Avoid using momentum; focus on a controlled and steady motion.
3. Start with a lighter weight to ensure proper form and avoid strain.

Active Muscles:
Primary: Abdominals (Rectus Abdominis)
Secondary: Shoulders (Deltoids), Hip Flexors (Iliopsoas)

Equipment:
Dumbbell

112. Dumbbell Russian Twist With Legs Floor Off

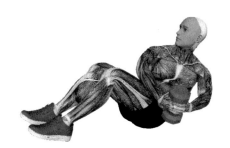 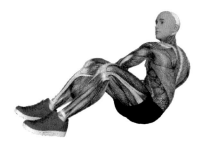

Instructions:

1. Sit on the floor with your knees bent and your feet lifted slightly off the floor, balancing on your glutes. Hold a dumbbell with both hands at chest level, keeping your back straight and core engaged.

2. Lean back slightly to form a V-shape with your torso and thighs, maintaining a straight spine.

3. Rotate your torso to the right, bringing the dumbbell beside your right hip while keeping your legs stable together.

4. Return to the center, then rotate your torso to the left, bringing the dumbbell beside your left hip. Continue alternating sides for the desired number of repetitions.

Tips:

1. Keep your legs stable and together to maintain balance.

2. Move slowly and with control to maximize muscle engagement.

3. Use a weight that allows you to maintain proper form throughout the exercise.

Active Muscles:
Primary: Obliques (External Obliques, Internal Obliques)

Secondary: Abdominals (Rectus Abdominis), Hip Flexors (Iliopsoas), Lower Back (Erector Spinae)
Equipment:
Dumbbell

113. Dumbbell Side Bend

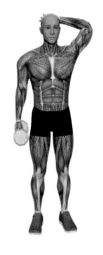

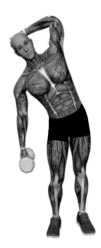

Instructions:

1. Stand with your feet shoulder-width apart, holding a dumbbell in your right hand with your arm fully extended by your side. Place your left hand behind your head.

2. Slowly bend to your right side at the waist, lowering the dumbbell towards the floor.

3. Bend as far as comfortably possible, feeling a stretch in your left oblique muscles.

4. Return to the starting position. Repeat for the desired repetitions, then switch to the left side.

Tips:

1. Avoid using momentum; focus on a slow and controlled movement.

2. Exhale as you bend to the side and inhale as you return to the starting position.

3. Keep your head and neck neutral, facing forward.

Active Muscles:
Primary: Obliques (External Obliques, Internal Obliques)
Secondary: Lower Back (Erector Spinae)

Equipment:
Dumbbell

114. Dumbbell Single Arm Starfish Crunch

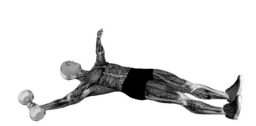 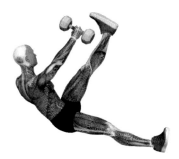

Instructions:

1. Begin by lying flat on your back with your arms and legs extended in a starfish position. Hold a dumbbell in your right hand and keep your left-hand firm on the floor.

2. Engage your core and lift your left leg and right arm simultaneously, aiming to touch the dumbbell to your left foot.

3. Reach as high as possible, squeezing your abdominal muscles at the top of the movement.

4. Lower your arm and leg back to the starting position in a controlled manner. Repeat for the desired repetitions, then switch to holding the dumbbell in your left hand and raising your right leg.

Tips:

1. Ensure your movements are slow and controlled to maximize muscle engagement.

2. Keep your non-working arm and leg extended on the floor for balance.

3. Focus on using your abs to lift your arm and leg, not your neck or shoulders.

Active Muscles:
Primary: Abdominals (Obliques, Rectus Abdominis)

Secondary: Hip Flexors (Iliopsoas), Shoulders (Deltoids), Chest (Pectoralis Major)
Equipment:
Dumbbell

115. Dumbbell Starfish Crunch Alternating

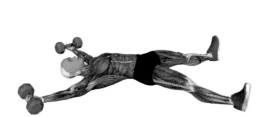 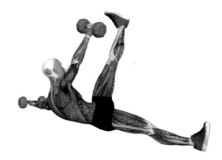

Instructions:
1. Begin by lying flat on your back with your arms and legs extended out in a starfish position, holding a dumbbell in each hand.
2. Simultaneously lift your right arm and left leg towards each other, crunching your torso and bringing the dumbbell towards your left foot.
3. Lower back down to the starting position with control.
4. Repeat the movement with your left arm and right leg, alternating sides for the desired number of repetitions.

Tips:
1. Perform the exercise in a controlled manner to maximize muscle engagement.
2. Avoid using momentum to lift your arms and legs; focus on the contraction of your core muscles.
3. Exhale as you lift your arm and leg, and inhale as you lower them back down.

Active Muscles:
Primary: Obliques (External Obliques, Internal Obliques)
Secondary: Abdominals (Rectus Abdominis), Hip Flexors (Iliopsoas), Shoulders (Deltoids)

Equipment:
Dumbbells

116. Dumbbell Straight Arm Crunch

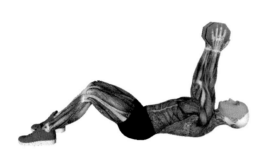 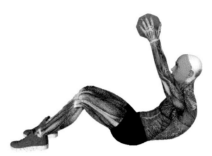

Instructions:

1. Begin by lying flat on your back with your knees bent and feet flat on the floor, holding a dumbbell with both hands extended straight above your chest.

2. Engage your core and lift your upper back off the floor, raising the dumbbell towards the ceiling as high as possible, while keeping your arms straight.

3. Lower your upper back, back to the floor with control, maintaining the arms extended above your chest. Repeat for the desired number of repetitions.

Tips:

1. Keep your arms straight and avoid bending your elbows during the movement.

2. Focus on reaching the dumbbell straight up rather than forward.

3. Exhale as you crunch up and inhale as you lower down.

Active Muscles:
Primary: Abdominals (Rectus Abdominis)
Secondary: Shoulders (Deltoids)

Equipment:
Dumbbell

117. Dumbbell Straight Arm Twisting Sit-Up

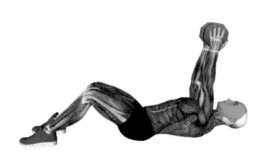 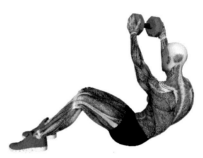

Instructions:

1. Begin by lying flat on your back with your knees bent and feet flat on the floor, holding a dumbbell with both hands extended straight above your chest.

2. Bend your core and lift your upper body off the floor, raising the dumbbell as high as possible towards the ceiling. As you crunch, twist your torso to the right, bringing the dumbbell towards your right side.

3. Lower your back to the floor with control, maintaining your arms extended above your chest. Repeat the movement, this time twisting to the left. Continue alternating sides for the desired number of repetitions.

Tips:

1. Keep your arms straight and avoid bending your elbows during the movement.

2. Use a weight that allows for proper form and control.

3. Exhale as you twist up and inhale as you lower down.

Active Muscles:
Primary: Obliques (External Obliques), Abdominals (Rectus Abdominis)
Secondary: Shoulders (Deltoids)

Equipment:
Dumbbell

118. Dumbbell Straight Leg Russian Twist

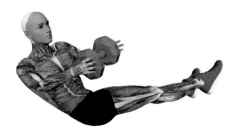 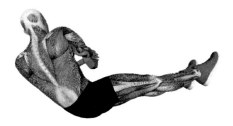

Instructions:
1. Sit on the floor with your legs extended straight just off the floor and hold a dumbbell with both hands close to your chest. Lean back slightly to engage your core, keeping your back straight.

2. Rotate your torso to the right, moving the dumbbell towards the floor beside your right hip, keeping your legs extended just off the floor.

3. Rotate your torso back to the center, bringing the dumbbell back to the center.

4. Continue rotating your torso to the left, moving the dumbbell towards the floor beside your left hip. Repeat for the desired number of repetitions, alternating sides.

Tips:
1. Avoid leaning back too far to prevent strain on your lower back.

2. Exhale as you twist to each side and inhale as you return to the center.

3. Keep your legs extended and together to maintain stability.

Active Muscles:
Primary: Obliques (External Obliques), Abdominals (Rectus Abdominis)

Secondary: Shoulders (Deltoids), Hip Flexors (Iliopsoas)
Equipment:
Dumbbell

119. Dumbbell V-Up

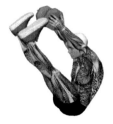

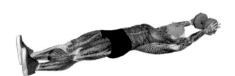

Instructions:

1. Begin by lying flat on your back with your legs extended straight and holding a dumbbell with both hands extended on the floor and arms fully extended.

2. Simultaneously lift your legs, upper body, and dumbbell off the floor, bringing your legs and arms together to form a V-shape.

3. Reach the dumbbell towards your feet, keeping your arms and legs straight.

4. Slowly lower your legs, upper body, and dumbbell back to the starting position. Repeat for the desired number of repetitions.

Tips:

1. Maintain straight arms and legs to maximize the effectiveness of the exercise.

2. Exhale as you lift into the V-up position and inhale as you lower back down.

3. Avoid jerking or using momentum; perform the movement in a controlled manner.

Active Muscles:
Primary: Abdominals (Rectus Abdominis)

Secondary: Hip Flexors (Iliopsoas)
Equipment:
Dumbbell

120. Over Head Weight Ab Crunch

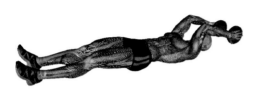 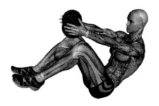

Instructions:

1. Begin by lying on your back with your legs straight on the floor. Hold a dumbbell with both hands, keeping your arms bent and close to your head and the floor.

2. Engage your core and lift your torso off the floor while bending your knees, raising them to your chest, and bringing the dumbbell close to your knees.

3. Lower your body back to the starting position with control. Repeat for the desired number of repetitions.

Tips:

1. Exhale as you crunch up and inhale as you lower back down.

2. Start with a lighter weight to master the form before progressing to heavier weights.

3. Perform the movement slowly and with control to maximize muscle engagement and avoid injury.

Active Muscles:
Primary: Abdominals (Rectus Abdominis), Hip Flexors (Iliopsoas)
Secondary: Shoulders (Deltoids), Upper Back (Trapezius)

Equipment:
Dumbbell

What Are Kettlebell Exercises?

Kettlebell exercises utilize a unique, ball-shaped weight with a handle that allows dynamic, swinging movements, making them distinct from traditional dumbbells or barbells. Kettlebells are highly versatile and can be used for a wide range of exercises, including swings, cleans, snatches, and Turkish get-ups. These movements engage multiple muscle groups, challenging co-ordination, balance, and core stability. Kettlebell workouts are known for combining strength training and cardiovascular conditioning, making them an effective tool for improving both endurance and muscle tone.

Why Use Kettlebell Exercises?

Kettlebell exercises provide a unique combination of strength, power, and endurance training. The dynamic nature of kettlebell movements, such as swings and snatches, engages the entire body, improving core stability, balance, and overall athleticism. Because of the constant movement and control required, kettlebells are excellent for boosting cardiovascular fitness while building muscle. Whether you're looking to improve functional strength or enhance athletic performance, kettlebells offer a flexible and effective option that can be adapted to all fitness levels.

121. Kettlebell Sit-Up Press

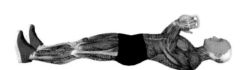 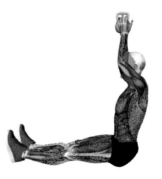

Instructions:

1. Begin by lying on your back with your legs straight on the floor, holding a kettlebell with both hands at your chest.

2. Lift your upper body off the floor until it is vertical to the floor, and then press the kettlebell overhead by extending your arms.

3. Lower the kettlebell back close to your chest.

4. Slowly lower your upper body back to the starting. Repeat for the desired number of repetitions.

Tips:

1. Use a controlled motion to lift and lower your upper body, avoiding any jerky movements.

2. Engage your core throughout the movement to maintain control and stability.

3. Choose a moderate weight for the kettlebell to ensure proper form and control.

Active Muscles:
Primary: Abdominals (Rectus Abdominis), Shoulders (Deltoids)

Secondary: Chest (Pectoralis Major), Triceps (Triceps Brachii), Core Muscles (Obliques)

Equipment:
Kettlebell

What Are Weight Plate Exercises?

Weight plate exercises involve using weight plates as a form of resistance during workouts. While weight plates are often used with barbells, they can also be used independently to create a variety of challenging exercises. Unlike machines that guide your movement, weight plates allow for a full range of motion and engage stabilizing muscles to control the weight. Weight plates can be used for various training goals, from building strength to improving balance and coordination, making them a versatile addition to any fitness routine.

Why Use Weight Plate Exercises?

Weight plate exercises offer unique advantages by targeting both large muscle groups and smaller stabilizing muscles that help with balance and control. This makes them particularly effective for building functional strength and enhancing overall muscle development. Since weight plates allow for greater movement flexibility, you can easily adjust the difficulty of your workout and target specific muscle groups. Whether you aim to increase strength, promote muscle hypertrophy, or improve athletic performance, weight plate exercises provide the versatility and challenge needed to progress at any fitness level.

122. Over Head Weight Sit Up

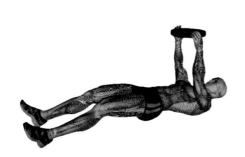

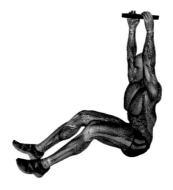

Instructions:

1. Begin by lying flat on your back with your legs slightly bent and your feet together. Hold a weight plate with both hands, extending your arms straight above your chest.

2. Engage your core and lift your upper body off the floor into a sitting position while extending the weight straight up.

3. As you sit up, ensure your back remains straight, and your chest is lifted, bringing your torso upright.

4. Lower your upper body back to the starting position with control. Repeat for the desired number of repetitions.

Tips:

1. Exhale as you crunch up and inhale as you lower back down.

2. Start with a lighter weight to master the form before progressing to heavier weights.

3. Perform the movement slowly and with control to maximize muscle engagement and avoid injury.

Active Muscles:
Primary: Abdominals (Rectus Abdominis)

Secondary: Shoulders (Deltoids), Upper Back (Trapezius)
Equipment:
Weight Plate

What Are Medicine/Weighted Ball Exercises?

Medicine ball exercises involve using a weighted ball to create resistance and enhance workouts. They are also known as weighted balls, are incredibly versatile, are available with and without handles, and can be used for a wide range of exercises targeting multiple muscle groups. Unlike machines that limit movement patterns, medicine balls allow for dynamic, full-range motion and engage stabilizing muscles. Medicine balls can be incorporated into various workout plans, from building power to improving coordination and explosive movements, making them an essential tool in any fitness routine.

Why Use Medicine/Weighted Ball Exercises?

Medicine ball exercises offer distinct benefits by challenging major muscle groups and smaller stabilizers, promoting balance, coordination, and functional strength. Additionally, because medicine balls come in various weights and sizes, they can be easily adapted to different fitness levels and specific training goals. Whether you want to increase strength, improve explosive power, or enhance core stability, medicine ball exercises provide the flexibility and intensity needed to advance your workout routine.

123. Crunch With Medicine Ball

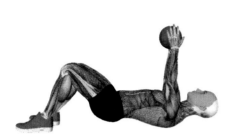 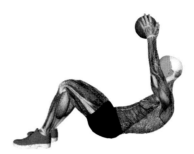

Instructions:

1. Lie on your back with your knees bent and feet flat on the floor, hip-width apart. Hold a medicine ball with both hands, extending your arms straight above your chest.

2. Lift your upper back off the floor by contracting your abdominal muscles.

3. Raise the medicine ball towards the ceiling as you perform the crunch, keeping your arms straight. Pause at the top of the movement for a second, squeezing your abs.

4. Slowly lower your upper body back to the starting position, keeping control of the movement. Repeat for the desired number of repetitions.

Tips:

1. Avoid using your neck muscles to lift your head; focus on using your abdominal muscles.

2. Ensure your feet remain flat on the floor and your knees stay bent at a consistent angle.

3. Keep the movement slow and controlled to maximize muscle engagement and prevent injury.

Active Muscles:
Primary: Abdominals (Rectus Abdominis)

Secondary: Shoulders (Deltoids), Upper Back (Trapezius)
Equipment:
Medicine Ball

124. Russian Twist Weighted Ball

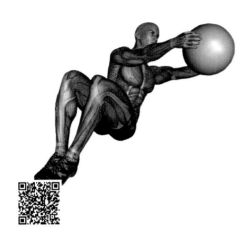 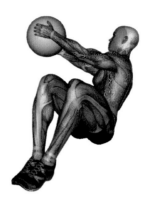

Instructions:
1. Sit on the floor with your knees bent and feet flat. Hold a weighted ball with both hands, keeping it opposite your chest with straight arms.
2. Lean back slightly, keeping your back straight.
3. Rotate your torso to the right, bringing the weighted ball towards the floor beside your hip.
4. Rotate your torso to the left, moving the weighted ball towards the floor beside your left hip. Repeat the twisting motion for the desired number of repetitions.

Tips:
1. Engage your core throughout the movement to maintain balance and stability.
2. Ensure your movements are smooth and controlled to maximize core engagement.
3. Focus on twisting from your torso, not just moving your arms from side to side.

Active Muscles:
Primary: Obliques (External Obliques), Abdominals (Rectus Abdominis)

Secondary: Shoulders (Deltoids), Hip Flexors (Iliopsoas)
Equipment:
Medicine Ball

CHAPTER 4

MACHINES

What Are Machine Exercises?

Machine exercises involve specialized gym equipment to guide your body through specific movements. These machines typically use pulleys, levers, and weight stacks to provide resistance, helping to target and isolate particular muscle groups. Examples include leg press machines, chest press machines, and cable machines, including Crossovers and Pulley Machines. Because the motion path is controlled, machine exercises are beneficial for ensuring proper form and reducing the risk of injury, making them an excellent option for beginners and those recovering from injury.

Why Use Machine Exercises?

Machine exercises offer several advantages, especially when targeting specific muscles without the need for balance or stabilizing muscles. Since the movement is guided, machines can help you maintain proper form and focus on the muscle being worked, which is beneficial for beginners or those working on improving an exercise technique. Additionally, machines provide a safer environment to lift heavier weights, particularly for those less experienced with free weights. They are excellent for building strength, muscle isolation, and gradually increasing resistance in a controlled setting.

125. Abdominal Crunches Machine

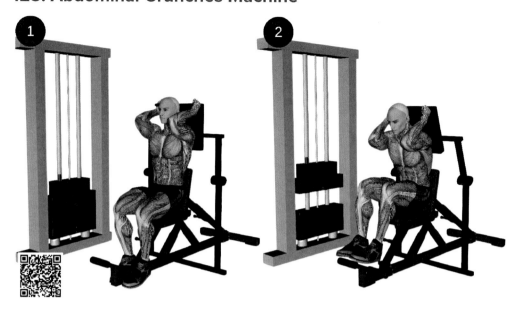

Instructions:

1. Adjust the seat and resistance to your desired settings on the abdominal crunch machine. Sit on the seat and position your feet securely on the footrests.

2. Grab the handles, ensuring your elbows are pointed forward.

3. Engage your core muscles and crunch your abdominals by pulling your upper body forward and curling your chest towards your knees.

4. Hold the crunch for a second, then slowly return to the starting position with control. Repeat for the desired number of repetitions.

Tips:

1. Exhale as you crunch and inhale as you return to the starting position.

2. Avoid using momentum; focus on engaging your abdominal muscles throughout the exercise.

3. Ensure your lower back remains in contact with the backrest of the machine.

Active Muscles:
Primary: Abdominals (Rectus Abdominis)
Secondary: Hip Flexors (iliopsoas)

Equipment:
Abdominal Crunch Machine

126. Cable Twist (Up-Down)

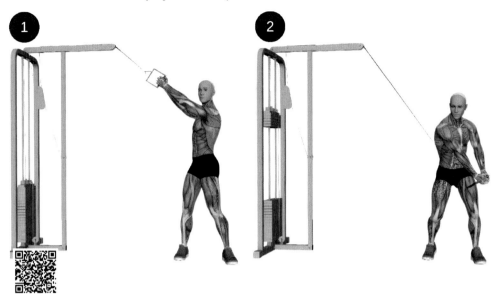

Instructions:

1. Stand sideways to the cable machine with your feet shoulder-width apart. Attach a handle to the high pulley and grasp it with both hands, arms extended diagonally along the cable.

2. Twist your torso down and across your body, pulling the handle down towards your opposite hip while keeping your arms straight.

3. Slowly return to the starting position with control.

4. Repeat for the desired number of repetitions, then switch sides.

Tips:

1. Perform the movement slowly and with control to maximize muscle activation and reduce injury risk.

2. Exhale as you twist away from the machine and inhale as you return to the starting position.

3. Minimize hip twisting to focus on engaging your obliques and core during the twist.

Active Muscles:
Primary: Obliques (External Obliques, Internal Obliques)
Secondary: Abdominals (Rectus Abdominis), Shoulders (Deltoids)

Equipment:
Cable Pulley Machine

127. Cable Twist

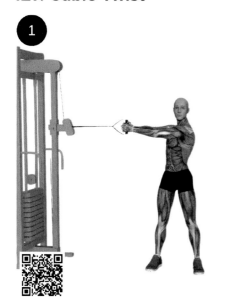

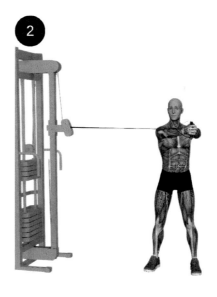

Instructions:

1. Stand sideways to the cable machine with your feet shoulder-width apart. Attach a handle to the pulley at shoulder height and grasp it with both hands, arms extended in front of you.

2. Twist your torso away from the machine, pulling the handle across your body while keeping your arms straight.

3. Slowly return to the starting position with control.

4. Repeat for the desired number of repetitions, then switch sides.

Tips:

1. Perform the movement slowly and with control to maximize muscle activation and reduce injury risk.

2. Exhale as you twist away from the machine and inhale as you return to the starting position.

3. Minimize hip twisting to focus on engaging your obliques and core during the twist.

Active Muscles:
Primary: Obliques (External Obliques, Internal Obliques)
Secondary: Abdominals (Rectus Abdominis), Shoulders (Deltoids)

Equipment:
Cable Pulley Machine

CHAPTER 5

RESISTANCE BANDS

What Are Resistance Band Exercises?

Resistance bands are flexible, stretchable rubber or latex bands that provide variable resistance during exercises. These bands come in different tension levels, allowing for a range of difficulty depending on your fitness level and specific movement. Resistance band exercises can target virtually every muscle group and can easily be adapted for strength training and rehabilitation. From banded squats to bicep curls, resistance bands offer a simple yet effective way to challenge your muscles without bulky equipment.

Why Use Resistance Band Exercises?

Resistance bands offer a unique combination of portability, versatility, and effectiveness, making them a great addition to any workout routine. They provide constant tension throughout the entire range of motion, which helps improve muscle activation and endurance. Resistance bands are also gentle on the joints, making them ideal for injury prevention and rehabilitation. Whether at home, traveling, or looking to add variety to your gym routine, resistance bands are an easy-to-use, lightweight option that can help improve strength, flexibility, and mobility at any fitness level.

128. Band Bicycle Crunch

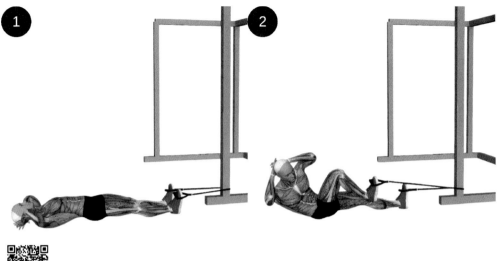

Instructions:

1. Lie on your back on the floor and secure a resistance band around both feet. Place your hands behind your head with your elbows pointing outward, and keep your legs extended straight.

2. Engage your core and lift your upper body off the floor. Bend your right knee towards your chest while twisting your torso to bring your left elbow towards your right knee.

3. Switch sides by bending your left knee towards your chest while bringing your right elbow towards your left knee, performing a pedaling motion.

4. Continue alternating sides in a controlled manner for the desired number of repetitions.

Tips:

1. Avoid pulling on your neck with your hands; use your abs to lift and twist your torso.

2. Ensure the resistance band is securely placed around your feet and on the equipment to avoid slipping.

3. Maintain a steady rhythm and focus on controlled movements rather than speed.

Active Muscles:
Primary: Obliques (External and Internal Obliques)

Secondary: Abdominals (Rectus Abdominis), Hip Flexors (Iliopsoas)
Equipment:
Resistance Bands

129. Band Decline Sit-Up

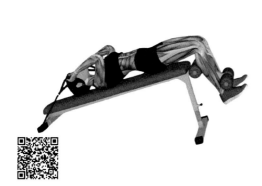

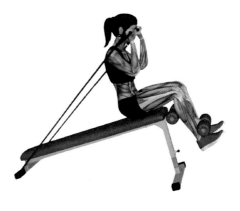

Instructions:

1. Secure the middle of the resistance band to a sturdy anchor point behind the headrest of a decline bench. Lie on the bench with your feet secured under the foot pads and hold one band handle in each hand, positioning the band over your shoulders.

2. Contract your abs and lift your upper body towards your knees, bringing your chest towards your thighs until you are in a seated position.

3. Slowly lower your upper body down the bench, maintaining control and tension in the band until your back rests on the bench.

4. Repeat for the desired number of repetitions.

Tips:

1. Ensure the resistance band is securely anchored behind the headrest to avoid slipping.

2. Exhale as you lift your upper body and inhale as you lower it back down.

3. Avoid pulling on the band with your arms; focus on using your abs to lift your body.

Active Muscles:
Primary: Abdominals (Rectus Abdominis)

Secondary: Hip Flexors (Iliopsoas)
Equipment:
Resistance Band, Decline Bench

130. Band Kneeling Crunch

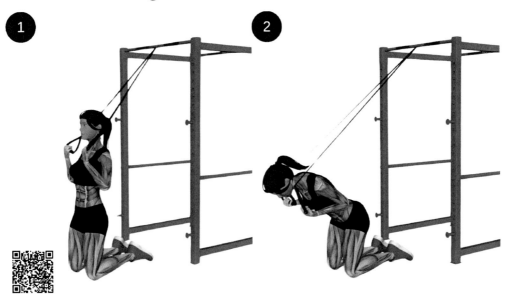

Instructions:

1. Secure the middle of the resistance band to a sturdy anchor point above head height. Kneel on the floor facing away from the anchor point, holding one handle of the band in each hand with your hands positioned at the sides of your head.

2. Engage your core and bend at the waist, bringing your elbows towards your knees in a controlled crunch motion.

3. Pause briefly at the bottom of the movement, ensuring a full contraction of your abdominal muscles.

4. Slowly return to the starting position with control. Repeat for the desired number of repetitions.

Tips:

1. Focus on using your abs to pull your torso down rather than your arms.

2. Ensure the resistance band is securely anchored to avoid slipping.

3. Exhale as you crunch down and inhale as you return to the starting position.

Active Muscles:
Primary: Abdominals (Rectus Abdominis)

Secondary: Obliques (External and Internal), Hip Flexors (Iliopsoas)
Equipment:
Resistance Band

131. Band Side Bend

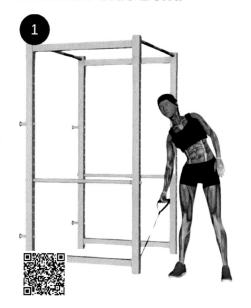
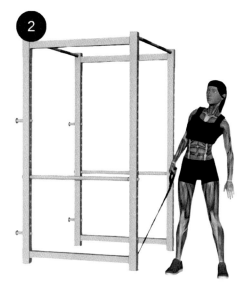

Instructions:

1. Anchor one end of the band at a low point of the equipment. Stand with your feet shoulder-width apart, your right side leaning to the anchor point, holding the other end of the resistance band in your right hand. Allow your left hand to hang by your side for counterbalance.

2. Contract your left obliques to bend at the waist to your left side until you are upright.

3. Return to the starting position with control.

4. Repeat the movement for the desired repetitions, then switch sides.

Tips:

1. Engage your core to help stabilize your body and prevent unnecessary movement.

2. Avoid bending forward or backward; focus on bending directly to the side.

3. Breathe steadily, exhaling as you bend to the side and inhaling as you return to the upright position.

Active Muscles:
Primary: Obliques (External Oblique, Internal Oblique)

Secondary: Abdominals (Rectus Abdominis), Lower Back (Erector Spinae)
Equipment:
Resistance Band

132. Diagonal Chop Cable

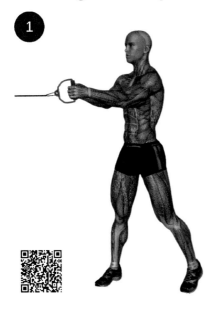

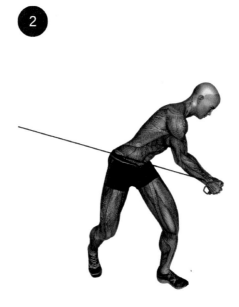

Instructions:

1. Anchor one end of the band at chest height. Stand with your right side facing the anchor point, with your feet shoulder-width apart, and grasp the handle with both hands. Extend your arms to hold the handle opposite your chest.

2. Pull the handle down and diagonally across your body, twisting your torso and pivoting your back foot to follow through. Bring the handle down towards the left side.

3. Slowly return to the starting position with control.

4. Repeat for the desired number of repetitions, then switch sides to work in the opposite direction.

Tips:

1. Perform the movement slowly and with control to maximize muscle activation and reduce injury risk.

2. Exhale as you pull the handle down and across your body, and inhale as you return to the starting position.

3. Use a lighter weight if needed to ensure proper form and gradually increase the resistance as you get stronger.

Active Muscles:
Primary: Obliques (External Oblique, Internal Oblique)

Secondary: Abdominals (Rectus Abdominis), Shoulders (Deltoids)
Equipment:
Resistance Band

133. High Resistance Band Kneeling Crunch

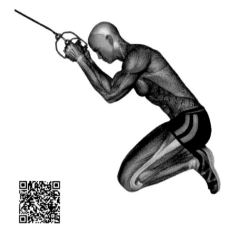

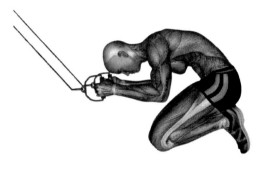

Instructions:

1. Attach a resistance band to a high anchor point. Kneel down facing the anchor point, holding the resistance band handles with both hands. Bend your arms at 90 degrees to bring your hands close to your face, palms facing each other.

2. Pull the resistance band down by crunching your torso towards your knees, bringing your elbows towards your thighs.

3. Slowly return to the starting position with control, keeping the tension on the band.

4. Repeat for the desired number of repetitions.

Tips:

1. Ensure your knees are firmly planted on the floor for stability.

2. Keep your hips stable and avoid using momentum.

3. Exhale as you crunch down and inhale as you return to the starting position.

Active Muscles:
Primary: Abdominals (Rectus Abdominis)

Secondary: Abdominals (Obliques), Hip Flexors (Iliopsoas)
Equipment:
Resistance Band

134. Lying Abs Resistance Band

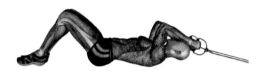 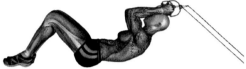

Instructions:

1. Lie on your back with your knees bent and feet flat on the floor. Attach the resistance band to a low anchor point behind your head and hold the handles with both hands, keeping your arms bent and handles close to your head.

2. Curl your upper body, bringing your elbows towards your knees while lifting your back off the floor.

3. Slowly lower your upper body back to the starting position with control.

4. Repeat for the desired number of repetitions.

Tips:

1. Exhale as you curl your torso up and inhale as you lower it back down.

2. Keep your feet flat on the floor for better stability.

3. Focus on engaging your abdominal muscles throughout the movement.

Active Muscles:
Primary: Abdominals (Rectus Abdominis)
Secondary: Abdominals (Obliques), Hip Flexors (Iliopsoas)

Equipment:
Resistance Band

CHAPTER 6

RESISTANCE LOOP BANDS

What Are Resistance Loop Band Exercises?

Resistance loop band exercises use looped elastic bands to create tension and resistance throughout various movements. These bands come in various resistance levels, from light to heavy, and can be used to target different muscle groups in upper and lower body workouts. Looped resistance bands provide constant tension throughout the entire movement, making them suitable for strength training, muscle activation, and rehabilitation exercises. Resistance loop bands are lightweight, portable, and adaptable to any fitness routine, making them ideal for at-home workouts or on-the-go training.

Why Use Resistance Loop Band Exercises?

Resistance loop band exercises are beneficial for targeting smaller, often underdeveloped muscles, helping to improve balance, flexibility, and overall functional strength. Whether recovering from an injury, aiming to build muscle, or enhancing your mobility, resistance loop bands provide a safe, low impact, yet challenging way to progress in your fitness journey. Their versatility and portability make them perfect for anyone, from beginners to advanced athletes, looking to maximize their results with minimal equipment.

135. Resistance Band Lying Bent Knee Raise

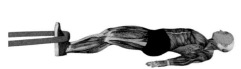 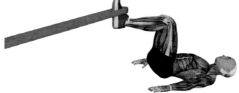

Instructions:

1. Attach the resistance loop band to a low anchor point and lie on your back with your knees bent and feet touching together. Wrap the other end of the loop resistance band over your feet. Place your arms on the floor by your sides.

2. Keep both legs straight and a few inches off the floor.

3. Slowly bend your knees and bring your legs up until your thighs are perpendicular to the floor and for a 90 degree.

4. Straighten your legs to the starting position with control and repeat for the desired number of repetitions.

Tips:

1. Focus on engaging your abdominals throughout the movement.

2. Avoid lifting your lower back off the floor; keep it pressed for the duration of the exercise.

3. Maintain a slight bend in your knee if necessary to reduce strain.

Active Muscles:
Primary: Abdominals (Rectus Abdominis)

Secondary: Hip Flexors (Iliopsoas), Quadriceps (Quadriceps Femoris)
Equipment:
Resistance Loop Band

136. Resistance Band Upper Body Dead Bug

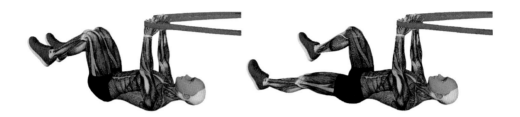

Instructions:

1. Lie flat on your back with your knees bent at a 90-degree angle, right above your hips. Attach two loop resistance bands at a low point, extending behind you.

2. Hold the end of each band in each hand, keeping your arms extended straight up towards the ceiling.

3. Lower your right leg towards the floor while keeping your left leg and arms in the starting position.

4. Repeat the movement with your left leg, alternating legs for the desired number of repetitions.

Tips:

1. Exhale as you lower your leg and inhale as you return it to the starting position.

2. Keep your lower back pressed into the floor to avoid strain.

3. Focus on engaging your core muscles throughout the movement.

Active Muscles:
Primary: Abdominals (Rectus Abdominis)

Secondary: Hip Flexors (Iliopsoas), Quadriceps (Quadriceps Femoris)
Equipment:
Resistance Loop Band

CHAPTER 7

SUSPENSION TRAINERS

What Are Suspension Trainer Exercises?

Suspension trainers, such as TRX systems, use straps with handles that can be anchored to a sturdy point to create a challenging, bodyweight-based workout. By adjusting the angle of your body and the straps, you can perform various exercises that engage multiple muscle groups at once. Suspension trainer exercises, like suspended push-ups or rows, leverage gravity and your body weight to build strength, improve flexibility, and enhance balance. The instability created by the suspension forces your core and stabilizer muscles to work harder, adding an extra layer of intensity to your routine.

Why Use Suspension Trainer Exercises?

Suspension trainers offer a dynamic and versatile way to improve functional strength and stability. Because they rely on your body weight and movement, they are highly adaptable to all fitness levels—you can easily modify exercises to make them more or less challenging by changing your body position. Suspension trainers also engage your core with almost every exercise, improving overall balance and coordination. Whether at home, in the gym, or outdoors, suspension trainers provide a portable and effective way to develop strength, flexibility, and stability with minimal equipment.

137. Suspension Trainer With Grips Abdominal Fallout

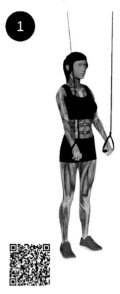

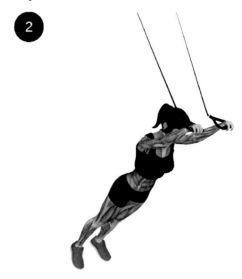

Instructions:

1. Adjust the suspension trainer handles to about waist height. Stand in front of the hanging handles with your feet shoulder-width apart and grasp the handles with your palms facing down.

2. Engage your core and lean forward, allowing your arms to extend overhead while maintaining a straight body line from head to heels.

3. Lower your body until your arms are fully extended above your head, feeling the tension in your core.

4. Pull your body back to the starting position by pulling your arms back to the starting position. Repeat for the desired number of repetitions.

Tips:

1. Breathe steadily: exhale as you lean forward and inhale as you return to the starting position.

2. Adjust the length of the suspension trainer straps to increase or decrease the difficulty of the exercise.

3. Keep your arms straight and avoid bending your elbows during the movement.

Active Muscles:
Primary: Abdominals (Rectus Abdominis)

Secondary: Upper Back (Trapezius, Rhomboids), Chest (Pectoralis Major), Shoulders (Deltoids)
Equipment:
Suspension Trainer with Grips

138. Suspension Trainer With Grips Hanging Knees To Elbows

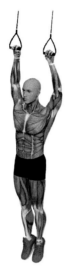

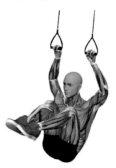

Instructions:

1. Adjust the suspension trainer handles to an overhead position. Grasp the handles with an overhand grip (palms facing forward) and hang with your arms fully extended and feet off the floor.

2. Engage your core and pull your knees towards your elbows, focusing on contracting your abdominal muscles.

3. Bring your knees as close to your elbows as possible while maintaining control and stability.

4. Slowly lower your legs back to the starting position with control. Repeat for the desired number of repetitions.

Tips:

1. Focus on using your abdominal muscles to lift your knees.

2. Breathe steadily: exhale as you lift your knees and inhale as you lower them.

3. Start with a smaller range of motion and gradually increase as your strength improves.

Active Muscles:
Primary: Abdominals (Rectus Abdominis)

Secondary: Hip Flexors (Iliopsoas), Shoulders (Deltoids)
Equipment:
Suspension Trainer with Grips

139. Suspension Trainer With Grips Hanging Straight Leg Hip Raise

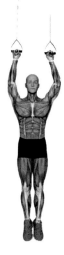

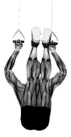

Instructions:

1. Adjust the suspension trainer handles to an overhead position. Grasp the handles with an overhand grip (palms facing forward) and hang with your arms fully extended and feet off the floor.

2. Engage your core and lift your knees towards the ceiling to hip height, then pull your hips up to raise your legs to chest height.

3. Slowly lower your legs back to the starting position with control, keeping your core engaged.

4. Repeat for the desired number of repetitions.

Tips:

1. Maintain a controlled motion to prevent swinging.

2. Focus on using your core muscles to lift your legs and hips, avoiding excessive use of your arms and legs.

3. Breathe steadily: exhale as you lift your legs and inhale as you lower them.

Active Muscles:
Primary: Abdominals (Rectus Abdominis)
Secondary: Hip Flexors (Iliopsoas), Shoulders (Deltoids)

Equipment:
Suspension Trainer with Grips

140. Suspension Trainer With Grips Pull Through

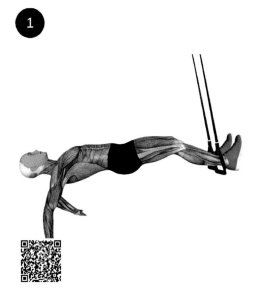

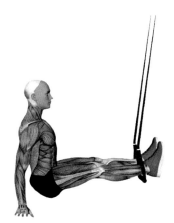

Instructions:

1. Adjust the suspension trainer handles to about knee height. Sit on the floor with extended legs and place your feet on the handles. Position your hands on the floor by your sides, fingers pointing forward.

2. Engage your core and press through your hands to lift your hips off the floor, coming into a reverse plank position. Your body should form a straight line from your head to your heels.

3. Lower your hips towards the floor with control, keeping your legs and arms straight. Stop just before your hips touch the floor.

4. Press through your hands and lift your hips to the reverse plank position. Repeat for the desired number of repetitions.

Tips:

1. Keep your core tight to maintain stability and prevent your hips from sagging.

2. Perform the movement with a steady and controlled tempo to maximize muscle engagement and prevent injury.

3. Breathe steadily: exhale as you lift your hips and inhale as you lower them.

Active Muscles:
Primary: Abdominals (Rectus Abdominis)

Secondary: Hip Flexors (Iliopsoas), Glutes (Gluteus Maximus), Lower Back (Erector Spinae)
Equipment:
Suspension Trainer with Grips

141. Suspension Trainer With Grips Reverse Ab Rollout

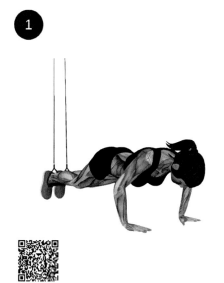

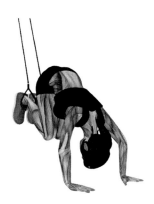

Instructions:

1. Adjust the suspension trainer handles to about knee height. Place your feet in the handles and assume a plank position with your hands slightly wider than shoulder width, placed directly under your shoulders, arms slightly bent, and body in a straight line from head to heels.

2. Engage your core and bend your knees to bring them to- wards your chest while lifting your hips upwards, creating an upside V position.

3. Continue bringing your knees towards your chest until your hips are fully bent and your knees are close to your chest.

4. Slowly extend your legs back to the starting plank position with control. Repeat for the desired number of repetitions.

Tips:

1. Breathe steadily: exhale as you bring your knees towards your chest, and inhale as you extend your legs back.

2. Start with a smaller range of motion and gradually increase as your strength and flexibility improve.

3. Keep your shoulders relaxed and avoid shrugging them towards your ears.

Active Muscles:
Primary: Abdominals (Rectus Abdominis)

Secondary: Hip Flexors (Iliopsoas), Shoulders (Deltoids)
Equipment:
Suspension Trainer with Grips

142. Suspension Trainer With Grips Supine Crunch

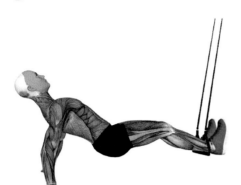 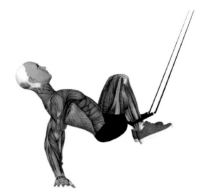

Instructions:

1. Adjust the suspension trainer handles to about knee height. Sit on your hips with your heels in the handles and legs extended straight and place your arms by your sides for support.

2. Engage your core and lift your hips off the floor while keeping your legs straight.

3. Curl your knees towards your chest and stop just before your knees touch your chest.

4. Slowly bring your legs back to the starting position. Repeat for the desired number of repetitions.

Tips:

1. Keep your core tight to maximize muscle engagement and prevent your back from arching

2. Start with a smaller range of motion and gradually increase as your strength improves.

3. Incorporate this exercise into your routine for a comprehensive core workout..

Active Muscles:
Primary: Abdominals (Rectus Abdominis)

Secondary: Hip Flexors (Iliopsoas), Shoulders (Deltoids), Lower Back (Erector Spinae)
Equipment:
Suspension Trainer with Grips

CHAPTER 8

AB ROLLER WHEEL

What Are Ab Roller Wheel Exercises?

Ab roller wheel exercises utilize a small wheel with handles on each side. As you roll the wheel forward and backward, you engage your abdominals, obliques, lower back, and even upper body muscles like the chest, shoulders, upper back, and arms. The ab roller wheel effectively builds core strength and stability while promoting balance and coordination. Common exercises include the traditional ab wheel rollout, extending your body forward while controlling the movement.

Why Use Ab Roller Wheel Exercises?

Ab roller wheel exercises provide an intense challenge for the entire core, requiring you to use both strength and control to maintain proper form throughout the movement. Unlike traditional crunches, the ab roller targets deep core muscles, helping to develop overall core stability and reduce the risk of lower back injuries. This tool strengthens your abs and improves your posture and functional strength, making it an essential addition to any fitness routine. Whether you want to increase core strength, build muscle definition, or enhance your overall body control, the ab roller wheel offers a powerful, compact solution to achieve those goals.

143. Ab Wheel All The Way Out

 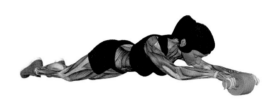

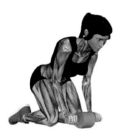

Instructions:

1. Start by kneeling on a mat with the ab wheel placed on the floor in front of you, holding it with both hands. Ensure your arms are extended and your back is straight.

2. Roll the ab wheel forward, extending your body into a straight line while keeping your core engaged and your hips slightly extended backward.

3. Roll the ab wheel back to the starting position, using your core muscles to control the movement and maintain stability.

4. Repeat the movement, extending fully and returning to the starting position each time.

Tips:

1. Keep your core muscles engaged throughout the exercise to protect your lower back and maintain stability.

2. Perform the movement slowly and with control, avoiding using momentum to maximize muscle engagement.

3. Ensure your hips are slightly extended backward when rolling out to maintain proper form and prevent lower back strain.

Active Muscles:
Primary: Abdominals (rectus abdominis)

Secondary: Hip Flexors (iliopsoas), Shoulders (deltoids)
Equipment:
Ab Roller Wheel

144. Ab Wheel Halfway Out

1

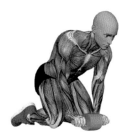

2

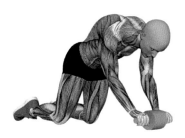

Instructions:

1. Start by kneeling on a mat with the ab wheel placed on the floor in front of you, holding it with both hands. Ensure your arms are extended and your back is straight.

2. Roll the ab wheel forward, extending your body halfway while keeping your core engaged and your hips slightly extended backward.

3. Roll the ab wheel back to the starting position, using your core muscles to control the movement and maintain stability.

4. Repeat the movement, extending halfway and returning to the starting position each time.

Tips:

1. Keep your core muscles engaged throughout the exercise to protect your lower back and maintain stability.

2. Perform the movement slowly and with control, avoiding using momentum to maximize muscle engagement.

3. Ensure your hips are slightly extended backward when rolling out to maintain proper form and prevent lower back strain.

Active Muscles:
Primary: Abdominals (rectus abdominis)

Secondary: Hip Flexors (iliopsoas), Shoulders (deltoids)
Equipment:
Ab Roller Wheel

145. Ab Wheel Plank

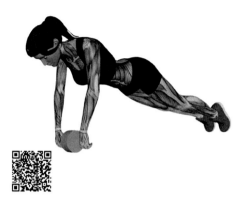

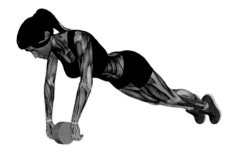

Instructions:

1. Start by kneeling on a mat with the ab wheel placed on the floor in front of you, holding it with both hands. Ensure your arms are extended and your back is straight.

2. Roll the ab wheel forward until your body is in a plank position, with your arms extend-ed and your body forming a straight line from head to knees.

3. Hold the plank position for as long as required, keeping your core engaged and your body stable.

4. Roll the ab wheel back to the starting position.

Tips:

1. Keep your spine neutral and avoid letting your lower back sag. This helps protect your spine and ensures proper form.

2. Focus on engaging your entire core, including your ab-dominals, obliques, and lower back, to maintain stability.

3. Roll out and back in with con-trolled movements to maxi-mize muscle engagement and minimize the risk of injury.

Active Muscles:
Primary: Abdominals (rectus abdominis)

Secondary: Obliques (external and internal obliques), Hip Flexors (iliopsoas)
Equipment:
Ab Roller Wheel

146. Ab Wheel Pulses

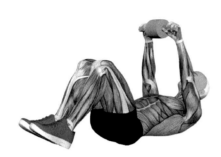

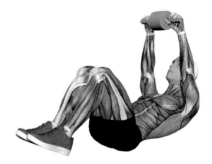

Instructions:

1. Start by lying on the floor with your arms extended overhead, holding the ab wheel with both hands.

2. Engage your core by lifting your upper body off the floor, performing a slight crunch while keeping your arms extended and the ab wheel overhead.

3. Perform small pulsing crunches, lifting and lowering your upper body slightly off the floor while maintaining tension in your core.

4. Continue the pulsing movement for the desired number of repetitions, keeping your arms extended and the ab wheel steady.

Tips:

1. Keep your movements small and controlled to maintain tension on your core muscles.

2. Focus on maintaining a neutral spine and avoiding any strain on your neck by using your core to lift your upper body.

3. Breathe steadily, exhaling as you lift into the crunch and inhaling as you lower back down.

Active Muscles:
Primary: Abdominals (rectus abdominis)

Secondary: Obliques (external and internal obliques)
Equipment:
Ab Roller Wheel

147. Ab Wheel Right Out

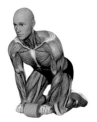

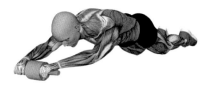

Instructions:
1. Start by kneeling on a mat with the ab wheel placed on the floor in front of you. Hold it with both hands. Ensure your arms are extended and your back is straight.
2. Roll the ab wheel forward to the right, extending your body into a partial straight line while keeping your core engaged and your hips slightly extended backward.
3. Roll the ab wheel back to the starting position, using your core muscles to control the movement and maintain stability.
4. Repeat the movement, rolling out to the right and returning to the starting position each time.

Tips:
1. Avoid overextending and roll out only as far as you can maintain control. Overextending can place unnecessary strain on your lower back and shoulders.
2. Breathe steadily. Inhale as you roll out and exhale as you roll back in. Proper breathing helps maintain core engagement and stability.
3. Ensure your hips are slightly extended backward when rolling out to maintain proper form and prevent lower back strain.

Active Muscles:
Primary: Abdominals (rectus abdominis), Obliques (external and internal obliques)

Secondary: Hip Flexors (iliopsoas), Shoulders (deltoids)
Equipment:
Ab Roller Wheel

Ab Roller Wheel

148. Ab Wheel Take It Or Leave It

1

2

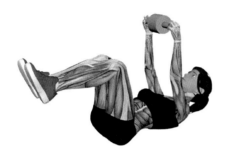
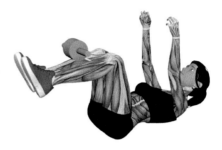

Instructions:

1. Lie on your back with your legs bent at 90 degrees and your feet off the floor, forming a table-top position. Hold the AB wheel overhead with both hands, keeping your arms straight.

2. Engage your core and lift your chest towards your knees to perform a crunch, bringing the AB wheel towards your shins.

3. Gently place the AB wheel on your shins and lower your upper body back to the floor, keeping your legs in the tabletop position.

4. Perform another crunch, reaching up to grab the AB wheel from your shins and then lower your upper body back to the floor. Repeat for the desired number of repetitions.

Tips:

1. Ensure your legs remain bent at 90 degrees and your shins parallel to the floor through-out the exercise.

2. Avoid using momentum to lift your upper body; focus on us-ing your abdominal muscles.

3. Perform the exercise on a comfortable, non-slip surface to ensure safety and reduce discomfort.

Active Muscles:
Primary: Abdominals (Rectus Abdominis)

Secondary: Hip Flexors (Iliopsoas)
Equipment:
Ab Roller Wheel

149. Reverse Ab Wheel Rollout

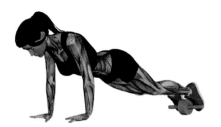
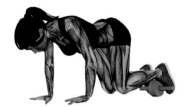

Instructions:
1. Begin in a plank position with your hands on the floor, arms straight, and the ab roller set under your feet. Your legs should be straight back, forming a straight line from head to heels.
2. Engage your core and slowly roll the ab roller towards your hands, keeping your legs straight. Continue rolling until your thighs are vertical to the floor.
3. Hold the position briefly, ensuring your core is tight and your back is straight.
4. Roll the ab roller back to the starting position with control, maintaining a straight line with your body. Repeat for the desired number of repetitions.

Tips:
1. Breathe steadily, exhaling as you roll the roller towards your hands and inhaling as you return to the starting position.
2. Avoid arching your back; maintain a neutral spine to prevent strain on your lower back.
3. Start with a small range of motion if you are new to this exercise, gradually increasing the distance as you build strength.

Active Muscles:
Primary: Abdominals (Rectus Abdominis)
Secondary: Shoulders (Deltoids), Quadriceps (Quadriceps Femoris)
Equipment:
Ab Roller Wheel

150. Standing Ab Wheel Rollout

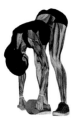
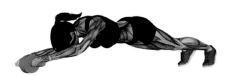

Instructions:

1. Stand with your feet shoulder-width apart, holding an ab wheel with both hands. Engage your core and maintain an upright posture.

2. Bend at your hips and knees to lower the ab wheel to the floor in front of your feet. Keep your arms extended and your back straight.

3. Slowly roll the ab wheel forward, extending your body into a plank position.

4. Roll the ab wheel back towards your feet, bending at your hips and knees to return to the starting position. Repeat for the desired number of repetitions.

Tips:

1. Perform the movement slowly and with control to maximize muscle activation and reduce injury risk.

2. Breathe steadily throughout the exercise, exhaling as you roll out and inhaling as you return.

3. Keep your back straight and avoid sagging or arching your lower back.

Active Muscles:
Primary: Abdominals (Rectus Abdominis)

Secondary: Shoulders (Deltoids), Quadriceps (Quadriceps Femoris)
Equipment:
Ab Roller Wheel

151. Wheels To Heaven

 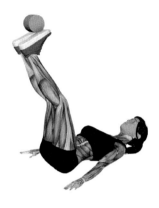

 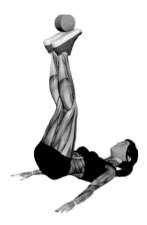

Instructions:

1. Lie on your back with your legs straight together and your arms resting by your sides. Position an ab roller between your heels.

2. Lift your legs towards the ceiling, keeping them slightly bent, holding the ab roller securely between your heels.

3. Engage your core and push your legs upward, raising your hips high off the floor.

4. Slowly lower your hips back down while keeping your legs up. Repeat for the desired number of repetitions.

Tips:

1. Start with a smaller range of motion if you are new to the exercise and gradually increase it as you gain strength.

2. Breathe steadily: exhale as you lift your legs and hips, and inhale as you lower them back down.

3. Avoid using momentum to lift your hips; focus on using your abdominal muscles.

Active Muscles:
Primary: Abdominals (Rectus Abdominis)

Secondary: Hip Flexors (Iliopsoas), Lower Back (Erector Spinae)
Equipment:
Ab Roller Wheel

152. Wheels To Toes

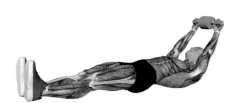

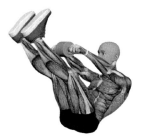

Instructions:
1. Lie on your back with your legs straight together, and your arms extended diagonally overhead, holding an ab roller.

2. Lift your legs towards the ceiling, keeping them straight, and simultaneously raise the ab roller towards your toes, lifting your upper back off the floor.

3. Slowly lower your legs and the ab roller back down to the starting position, stopping just before they touch the floor.

4. Repeat the movement for the desired number of repetitions.

Tips:
1. Use a mat or soft surface to support your back and prevent discomfort.

2. Ensure your lower back stays in contact with the floor when your legs are lowered.

3. Start with a smaller range of motion if you are new to the exercise and gradually increase it as you gain strength.

Active Muscles:
Primary: Abdominals (Rectus Abdominis)
Secondary: Hip Flexors (Iliopsoas), Shoulders (Deltoids)

Equipment:
Ab Roller Wheel

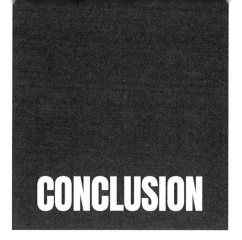

CONCLUSION

Congratulations! By completing this guide, you've taken significant steps toward strengthening your core and enhancing your overall fitness. But remember, fitness is a journey, not a destination. Whether you've reached a specific goal or are just beginning to see the results of your hard work, keep challenging yourself to improve daily.

The exercises and techniques in this book are just the foundation. As you continue your fitness journey, use this guide as a reference to expand your workouts, try new exercises, and push your limits. Fitness is about consistency and progress, and with dedication, the results will follow.

Remember, no matter where you are on your fitness path, every rep, every set, and every day you dedicate to self-improvement brings you closer to your goals. You have the tools now—keep going, and you will continue to achieve great things!

ACKNOWLEDGMENTS

Thank you for choosing **The Ultimate Exercise Guide: Abdominals Edition**. This book has been three years in the making—a journey filled with countless hours of hard work, perseverance, and determination to bring this project and our entire business to life. What started as a simple idea has grown into a comprehensive resource, and it would not have been possible without the support and dedication of so many people.

First and foremost, I want to express my deepest gratitude to the incredible team at **N.C.A. HEALTH & WELLNESS LTD**. Despite the challenges we've faced, your commitment to our vision has been nothing short of inspiring. Together, we've worked through long nights, difficult moments, and endless revisions to ensure that this book and our business could offer the very best to our readers and clients.

To the talented illustrators and designers, thank you for bringing our ideas to life with such creativity and precision. Your expertise has transformed this guide into a visually engaging and easy-to-follow guide.

Finally, to you, the reader, thank you for trusting this guide and our work. Your support helps us continue to grow, create more content, and expand our offerings. We've built this business with you in mind, and your dedication to your fitness journey drives us to keep going.

This book and business are the results of years of hard work, and I'm grateful to everyone who has contributed to them.

Thank you all.

-

Nicolas Andreou

Stay Connected

We'd love to hear about your progress! Please consider leaving a review to let others know how this guide has helped you in your fitness journey. Your feedback helps us improve and allows others to find valuable resources like this.

For more exercises, video tutorials, and fitness content, be sure to check out ExerciseAnimatic.com. Don't forget to use the code **'IBOUGHTYOURBOOK'** to get a 20% discount on our **Ultimate Bundle** or individual exercise videos on your first order.

Thank you for supporting our work and being part of our growing fitness community. Keep pushing your limits, and we'll be here to support you every step of the way.

What's Next?

This is just the beginning! We are continuously working on expanding our exercise library and creating more resources to help you achieve your fitness goals. Stay tuned for more volumes in the **Ultimate Exercise Guide** series, covering other muscle groups.

Made in the USA
Las Vegas, NV
17 November 2024

3edb2e8d-b566-49bb-84c0-249db621e91dR01